ISBN-13: 978-1452801421

ISBN-10: 1452801428

Original Printing by Lulu Press, 2009

East Meets West:
An Integrative Approach to
Managing Overuse Injury

Dr. Diane Gross, DOM (NM), L.Ac., Dipl. OM, HLC

Special Thanks

I am immensely grateful for the generous support of those who assisted me during various stages of writing this book. I would like to thank my wonderful husband, Richard, for his encouragement, his staunch love, and for his faith in me - as well as for the many, many hours he spent formatting this book. I appreciate the amazing editing by my son and colleague in Oriental medicine, Mark Gross, L.Ac. A special thanks to Dr. Michael Feuerstein, for everything he taught me about preventing and managing overuse injury from a western medical perspective. I am also immensely grateful to my instructors at Southwest Acupuncture College who taught me so much about treating overuse injury from an Oriental medical perspective. Thank you all.

Table of Contents

Introduction

Chapter 1- Overuse Injury

Chapter 2- Predisposing Factors to Overuse Injury

Chapter 3- Ergonomics and Overuse

Chapter 4- Developing Low Risk Ergonomics

Chapter 5- Rest and Recovery Time

Chapter 6- Exercise to Reduce Risk of Overuse

Chapter 7- Stress Management

Chapter 8- Pain Management

Chapter 9- A Plateful of Pain - or Energy?

Chapter 10- Self Care Using Acupressure and Self-Massage

Chapter 11- The Yin and Yang of Time

Chapter 12- Work Stations

Chapter 13- Making Your Body Your Ally

Note from the Author:

In writing this book I considered the question of whether I should write using the pronouns "you" and "your" or the more general pronouns of "we" and "our." My concern was that using the more direct terms of "you" and "your" might sound like I was lecturing, or even preaching. Yet the use of "we" and "our" often felt like the message of personal empowerment and individual responsibility for health and choices got lost. For example, the phrase "making *your* body your ally" has a very different feel to it than "making *our* bodies our allies." For me the first phrase is much more personal and powerful. As a result, I decided to use "you" and "your." My hope is that you, the reader, will find the information instrumental in helping you establish a long, enjoyable and healthy life and career.

Introduction

Pain is often seen as an unavoidable professional liability by individuals working in professions requiring repetitive movements. Symptoms of overuse in these types of professions are commonplace. In fact, according to the Bureau of Labor Statistics, U.S. Department of Labor, injuries from repetitive motion, or overuse, continue to be the cause of the highest median days away from work for all private industries (20 days). Musculoskeletal disorders accounted for 29 percent of all workplace injuries *requiring time away from work* in 2007.[2] This number doesn't include injuries *not* requiring time away from work, thus it appears this statistic may be just the tip of the iceberg. It is considered to be the leading reason for worker's compensation claims and lost wages in the United States today.

It is vital to employ prevention strategies designed to reduce the risk of overuse symptoms, as well as to respond pro-actively to symptoms should they arise. If you believe pain and your profession go "hand-in-hand," you are less likely to take action to mitigate the cause of your pain. I think *a much more useful approach is to recognize pain for what it is – a signal from your body that something needs attention.* Pain is an extremely important feedback mechanism, and it is important to pay careful attention to its message and to respond accordingly.

I originally became involved in working with people experiencing overuse injury in 1990 while working as a sign language interpreter at the National Technical Institute of Technology (NTID). NTID's interpreting department was in crisis due to the number of work related injuries interpreters were experiencing. Out of 65 staff interpreters, 73% were receiving some form of work related accommodation due to symptoms. This was, of course, a major institutional crisis, in addition to the individual crisis for each person involved.

As a result of an intensive study conducted by NTID and The Center of Occupational Rehabilitation, part of the University of Rochester Medical Center, significant predisposing factors were identified in those interpreters working with pain as compared to those working with little or no pain.[4, 5]

Following this study, NTID administration asked me to lead in the development of training materials for interpreters on the prevention and management of interpreting related injury. I accepted the challenge and was privileged to serve as project coordinator and senior writer in the development of these materials. This project required five years of working with experts in the fields of exercise physiology, occupational medicine, physical therapy, chiropractic, acupuncture, psychology, interpreting, and interpreter education.

During this time, I had the opportunity to be trained in the identification and remediation of high-risk ergonomics. I have been able to successfully apply these principles to both the interpreting field and other high risk professions because the principles are the same. For almost twenty years, I've been privileged to work with people all over the United States.

Eventually, I went back to school for Oriental medicine. I became licensed as a Doctor of Oriental Medicine (DOM) in New Mexico, and a Licensed Acupuncturist (L.Ac.) in North Carolina. The materials that follow will utilize my expertise as a doctor of oriental medicine and acupuncturist, as well my ergonomic experience.

In this book, prevention and management of overuse injury will be explored from a multi-dimensional and often holistic perspective. Issues of ergonomics, scheduling, exercise, stress management, pain management, nutritional interventions, and self-care, including the use of acupressure and self-massage, will be addressed.

While this book can be helpful to those who are dealing with minor overuse symptoms, or for those seeking a sound preventative program, it is not meant to replace medical care for substantial, acute and/or chronic issues. It is also not meant to replace ergonomic diagnostic feedback by a qualified professional.

Chapter 1

Overuse Injury

Over the years various terms and acronyms have been utilized to describe the symptoms of injury due to "overuse." Some of the more common ones are Repetitive Motion Injury (RMI), Repetitive Strain Disorder (RSD), Overuse Syndrome, and Cumulative Trauma Disorder (CTD). Overuse, for the purposes of this book, refers to a variety of disorders typically associated with, but not limited to, overuse, repetitive movements, poor ergonomics and/or insufficient rest or recovery time. However, there are a number of things beside repetitive movements that can substantially impact your risk of injury. For example, working in a cold room may potentially increase the risk of injury as much as the repetitive motions involved while engaged in a specific task. There are other additional factors, such as anatomical or physiological predispositions, that may play a significant role in the development of an overuse injury that will be discussed.

Overuse injury is related to the muscles, as well as nerves, tendons, ligaments, the neurovascular system and bones. Some of the more common ones are muscle soreness, tendonitis, tenosynovitis, carpal tunnel syndrome, De Quervains syndrome, and nerve impingement at various locations in the upper extremity. A short definition of each of these disorders is as follows:[6]

- ♣ **Muscle soreness:** Muscle soreness due to muscle exertion. This is often a result of lactic acid accumulation in the muscle or inflammation.

- ♣ **Tendonitis:** Inflammation of a tendon. This often happens as a result of repeated stress placed on the tendon due to overuse or poor ergonomics.

- ♣ **Tenosynovitis:** Inflammation of the synovial membrane of a tendon. One of the most common areas affected is the wrist. Often this is related to excessive hand/wrist flexion.

- ♣ **Carpal Tunnel Syndrome (CTS):** Compression of the median nerve as it passes through the carpal tunnel in the wrist. There are many factors that can lead to CTS, including inflammation of the tendons in the carpal tunnel and a reduction in carpal tunnel space due to anatomical or physiological changes (e.g. bone spur, arthritis, overuse, hormonal imbalances, etc.).

- ♣ **De Quervain's Syndrome:** A type of tenosynovitis affecting the abductor muscles of the thumb and the side of the wrist.

- ♣ **Nerve Impingement:** Trapped, impinged or compressed nerves possibly due to anatomical or physiological changes.

Types of Symptoms Associated with Overuse: Usually the first symptom associated with overuse is an achy sensation. If it is not addressed it can worsen. The most common types of *initial* symptoms related to overuse are:

- ♣ Aching

- ♣ Redness and swelling of affected area

- ♣ Paresthesia, an abnormal prickling, tingling, burning, or crawling sensation on the skin.

- ♣ Numbness and loss of sensation

- ♣ Coldness

- ♣ Color changes (due to circulation problems)

- ♣ Reduction in range of motion (ROM)

- ♣ Joint impairment, including locking, clicking, triggering, popping, etc.

- ♣ Weakness, with accompanying reduction in ability to grip and hold things

It is important to know if the symptoms you are experiencing are serious in nature, and require medical intervention, or if they simply require a little extra rest and self-care.

You certainly want to make sure you get medical attention if that is indeed what is required. At the same time, with rising medical costs, if medical intervention is truly not necessary it can be helpful to know that as well! While there is no way that I can give "fool proof" or definitive advice, especially without the benefit of conducting a physical examination, there are some guidelines that can be helpful.

- **It is significant to determine if the pain is sudden or gradual.** A sudden onset of pain may point to an acute or traumatic cause. If you experience a sudden onset of pain, it is important to seek medical attention since this could indicate a soft tissue tear or injury of a more substantial nature. Gradual onset pain is often less serious, but still should be addressed in order to prevent worsening over time.

- **The quality of pain can help identify the source of the problem and determine if medical attention is warranted.** Dull, throbbing, or aching pain is often due to overuse or poor ergonomics. Generally this type of pain indicates muscle or soft tissue problems. In oriental medicine, different types of pain are important aspects of differential diagnosis.

  o Muscle or soft tissue problems due to overuse can often be resolved simply by resting. Conversely, sharp pain - especially with movement - may be a sign of severe muscle spasms, or even a ligament, tendon, or muscle tear.

  o Burning, radiating and shooting pain, and/or tingling and numbness often indicate nerve involvement.

  o Nerve involvement or any ligament, tendon or muscle tear requires medical attention.

- **If the same movement always produces the same pain in the same place on the body, it probably indicates that there is a specific injury that needs to be addressed, or that the activity may exacerbate the condition if continued.** This is an important consideration because continuing to work in ways that precipitated symptoms, *while experiencing pain* will only produce more of the same.

♣ **Whether the pain is localized or referred may be telling.** When I was in school for Oriental medicine my instructors would say "the injury is often *not* where it hurts." One instructor explained it with the adage, "It's not usually the bully on the playground that's the one complaining!" This is important because the goal is to remediate the *source* of the pain. Often you can know if the pain is referred or local, depending on if it is focal or diffuse. Focal pain tends to be caused by a problem in the local area. More diffuse pain tends to be referred from the actual area of injury. It can be helpful to look at a book or chart showing various "trigger points" on the body and the areas to which they refer pain.

♣ **If pain is coupled with other symptoms, it may indicate a more complex or serious condition.** It can also be indicative of a connection between the two areas of the body. For example, Carpal Tunnel Syndrome (CTS) frequently has its genesis in the shoulder/neck region, or even the elbow.

♣ **What helps improve symptoms and what causes them to worsen can be useful information.** There may be some joint or muscle dysfunction if movement makes it worse. If pain is worse with *passive* movement (i.e. someone else moves your arm for you and it hurts worse than when you move it yourself) that usually indicates ligament involvement. If pain shows no improvement with rest, medical attention should be sought. On the other hand, it is a positive sign if rest helps. If pain reappears quickly with resumed use, it could indicate the rest was insufficient, resumption of activity was too much and too fast, or it could mean that there is an underlying injury that needs to be addressed.

♣ **If the pain responds positively to the application of heat or ice, it may indicate inflammation.** I often recommend anti-inflammatory foods and herbs such as turmeric, ginger, bromelain, and fish oil in this instance. I do not advocate the ongoing use of ice as a therapeutic modality for a chronic condition. I will address this later in the book.

♣ **How long the pain lasts is an important consideration.** We all have experienced short-lived pain such as sore muscles from time to time, but if the pain is relentless or chronic it needs to be addressed.

In a nutshell, if symptoms are sudden in onset, severe, sharp in quality, coupled with other significant symptoms, don't improve with rest, or are easily exacerbated and reproduced, you should receive a medical assessment. If pain has a gradual onset, is not intense, has an aching or throbbing quality, subsides with rest and improves with ice or heat, then the injury is probably fairly benign. However, it is important to keep in mind that unless the initial symptoms are addressed the problem could become acute. Paying attention to your body empowers you with information. It allows you the opportunity to make more informed choices about your health.

Chapter 2
Predisposing Factors to Overuse

As depicted in Figure 1 below, there are a number of components that comprises a work task. These components may filter through a variety of predisposing factors that impact the risk of overuse injury.

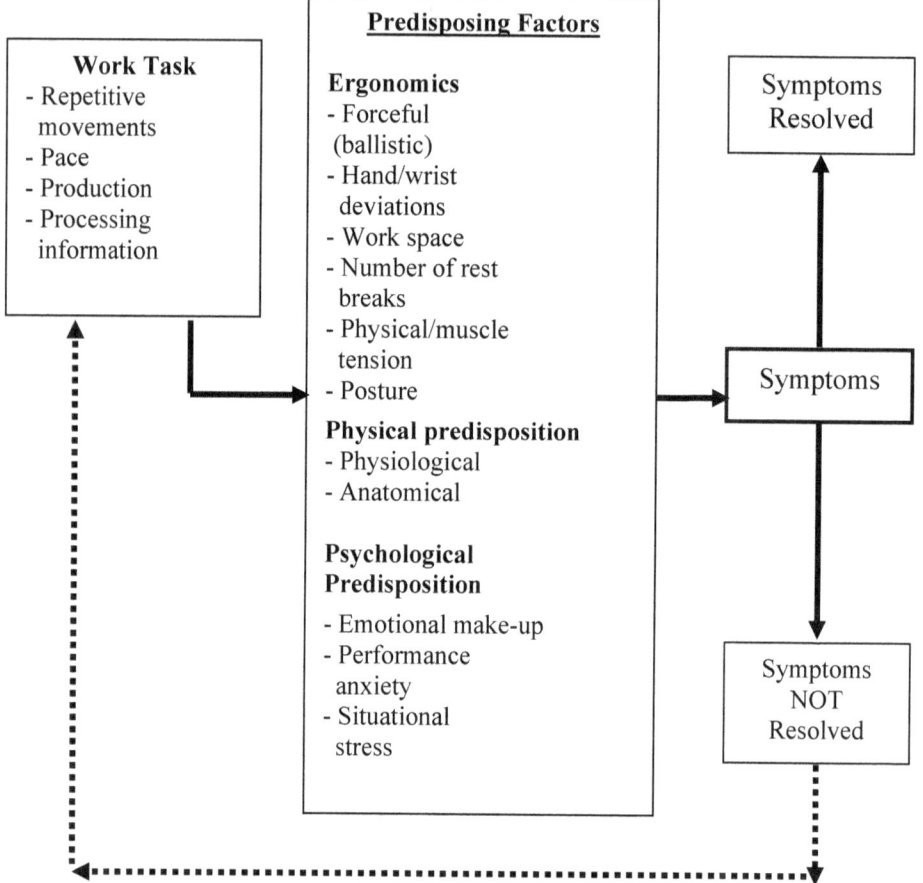

Figure 1: The Overuse Injury Cycle

While this is by no means a comprehensive list, it represents some of the essential elements of any work requiring repetitive motions, including:

- ♣ Repetitive Movements

- ♣ Pace Required to do the Work

- ♣ Production of Work

- ♣ Processing of Information

While the demands of the any work task may be impactful, the *significance* of the impact depends on the predisposing factors through which they are filtered. The greater the number of harmful filters, and the more severe the filters in question are – the greater the potential impact.

The predisposing filters through which the work can pass include:

Ergonomics and Body Mechanics: Chapter 3 will cover ergonomics extensively. It is an incredibly important aspect of staying healthy and a pivotal piece of the Overuse/Work task connection, one over which you can have control.[7]

Physical Predispositions: There are two basic categories of physical predispositions. They are anatomical and physiological.

Anatomical Predispositions: This refers to specific anatomical or structural concerns that may increase the risk of overuse injury as a result of additional stress placed on the body. These may include such things as:

- ♣ **Bone/spine abnormalities.** Examples include spinal subluxation, osteoporosis, bone spurs, etc.

- ♣ **Tendon/muscle/ligament abnormalities.** Examples include tendonitis, soft muscle injury, micro-tears, sprains, strains, spasms, etc.

- ♣ **Previous anatomical injuries or surgeries.** Examples include improperly healed broken bone, spinal fusion, pins or plates, etc.

Physiological Predispositions: A physiological predisposition can refer to a wide variety of physical factors that can impact the risk of overuse injury. These may include:

* **Physical muscle tension**. Muscle tension can be caused by several things:

  o **Emotional tension.** Science has demonstrated that there is indeed a mind-body connection. If you are feeling emotionally stressed, then you *will* experience physical muscle tension. It is not possible to separate the two. Chapter 8 will address the topic of emotional tension and stress management more fully.

  o **Learned muscle patterns.** Your muscles have 'muscle memory.' In other words, your muscles learn specific ways of functioning, or 'habits' based on your regular patterns of movement and ways in which you habitually hold your body. If you sit and stand with poor posture on a regular basis, your muscles learn to remember and reproduce this type of posture as a default position. If you live with a lot of emotional and physical stress, your muscles "learn" or habituate tension. This is one reason a daily practice of relaxation techniques can be so helpful. They can help you "unlearn" old, unhealthy patterns and develop new, healthier ones.

  o **Static loading.** Static loading occurs when you hold your muscles in an awkward or tense position for an extended period of time, leading to muscle tension and spasm. An example is constantly "holding" the shoulders up as opposed to down in a relaxed position. You may feel the result of static loading in your arms, neck, or back, depending on which muscles are being stressed.

* **Hormonal imbalances.** Examples include:

  o **Diabetes.** Diabetes is a disease in which the body is unable to produce or properly utilize insulin. Insulin is a required for the conversion of food into the energy necessary for daily life. The function of the entire body and its ability to do work is compromised when insulin levels are not in balance.

- o **Thyroid imbalances**. The thyroid regulates many functions in the body, including heart rate, digestion, physical growth, etc. If this gland, and the hormone it produces, is out of balance, muscle weakness and damage can result.

- o **PMS and pregnancy.** Many hormonal imbalances can occur around the menses and during pregnancy. One example that can impact the risk of overuse injury is the fluid retention that often occurs at these times. This fluid can cause tissue to swell and put pressure on nerves, especially in the carpal tunnel.

- ♣ **Fatigue.** Fatigue can play a significant role in your physiological response to work. Rest and recovery time are important aspects of living a balanced life style. Your body, mind, and spirit needs time to recoup from your busy schedule and life.

- ♣ **Impaired or insufficient sleep.** It is absolutely essential that you get enough quality sleep. Some experts believe that as much as 80% of your body's healing occurs during sleep. Deep, nourishing sleep is required if your body's cells are to fully recover from normal wear and tear, let alone heal from micro injuries that have resulted from overuse.

- ♣ **Poor nutrition.** A balanced diet is necessary to provide the foundation with which to nourish, energize and repair the body. When these foundational nutrients are unavailable to the body, the chance for injury increases. Additionally, there are foods that can actually assist in the healing process, and others that can hinder the body's attempts to heal. These will be discussed in Chapter 9 in greater detail.

- ♣ **Poor muscle strength, endurance and flexibility.** The level of your "fitness" impacts your risk of getting an overuse injury. It can be helpful to think of this in terms of "work capacity." Work capacity is that level of work that can be safely managed without risk of injury. If you are always working at, or very near, your work capacity in a field requiring repetitive motions, then your chance of injury is increased. The easiest way to reduce your risk of injury is to increase your work capacity. The result is the ability to perform the physical demands of tasks requiring repetitive movements with greater ease.

♣ **Poor general health.** Poor overall health may be due to some of the factors already discussed, or some other cause such as disease. Regardless of what those factors may be, if there are general health issues, then the risk of overuse injury may increase.

Psychological Predisposition:

When I first began working with people on preventing and managing overuse injury, I thought ergonomic predispositions were the most significant determining factors for overuse. After more than 17 years of teaching workshops and performing ergonomic diagnostics, I now believe that psychological predispositions are actually the most significant. It impacts the risk of injury at every level. It influences how you take care of yourself physically, how you approach your work, how you manage your pre-disposing factors, whether you advocate for yourself, and how you respond if you experience discomfort from your work. Here are some examples of psychological predispositions to overuse injury:

♣ **External locus of control:** An external locus of control means to approach life as if it happens *to* you. An *internal* locus of control acknowledges that your personal choices determine how you experience life. An external locus of control can set you up for injury.

For example, suppose your computer desk is much too high. You find yourself just peeking over the edge of the desk and must type with your elbows up by your ears. Obviously I am being a bit facetious, but there have been times I have been presented with a situation that is not so different from this scenario! If you have an external locus of control you may accept the situation as inevitable and do your best to "work with it." In doing so, you set yourself up for injury.

It is essential, professionally and personally, to have an internal locus of control. This will enable you to be resolute about what you need in order to do your work safely. An external locus of control would result in "sucking it up" and limping through the day regardless of resulting fatigue or pain levels. An internal locus of control would allow you to feel comfortable requiring some kind of accommodation that respects your physical safety needs and limitations. This could be requesting support, working for only part of the scheduled event, asking for breaks every hour, or for another option that doesn't place you at risk of injury.

If you are currently managing an existing injury, being externally focused can create a "why did this injury have to happen to me" mentality. A more helpful approach might be, "This happened. Now what do I need to do in order to help myself in the best way possible?" An external locus of control keeps you stuck; while an internal locus of control helps you find and follow through with empowering choices.

♣ **"Savior" mentality:** Sometimes people find themselves constructing their lives and schedules around their work demands – to their own detriment. Sentiments such as, "If I don't get this done, then it won't get done," and "I'm the only person who can do this," are not helpful.

This kind of thinking and acting can easily cause you to live from a martyr stance, and may result in personal injury. Choosing to take care of one's self is not something that society has always encouraged and valued. Sometimes it is seen as selfish or self-centered. And yet, do you really serve anyone if you function in ways that bring harm to your own self? Taking care of yourself enables you to remain healthy enough to serve and work in a balanced way.

Years ago I was personally dealing with an overuse injury working as a sign language interpreter in a college setting. The semester was only half over, but my pain levels were severe. There were no other interpreters available to replace me in the classes I was interpreting. I found myself struggling with feelings of guilt at the thought of taking the rest of the semester off - and yet I knew I desperately needed to take care of myself! I remember my supervisor wisely saying to me, "While it would be very unfortunate, the worse case scenario is that the student may have to take the class again, but you only have two arms to last you for the rest of your life. Take care of them. You will not ultimately be doing anyone a favor if you injure yourself to the point that you actually have to leave your field due to injury." I have never forgotten that feedback.

- ♣ **Stressful thinking:** When you engage in chronic stressful thinking it affects every bodily system. In addition to inhibiting blood circulation, upsetting your body's hormonal balance, and causing physical muscle tension, chronic stress can also affect the ability of your cells to receive nutrition from the food you eat! The cell receptors can actually get "hijacked" by the stress hormones. Obviously this impacts the ability of your body to repair and nourish itself.

  Additionally, when you engage in stressful thinking your cognitive abilities are compromised. This makes processing information more difficult, which in turn can create more physical stress. If you are already managing an overuse injury and must advocate for your own well-being, having full cognitive abilities would be important.

- ♣ **Perfectionism:** I think an "Achilles heel" of many people is demanding perfectionism in their life and work. This is not to imply that your goal should be anything less than producing work of the highest quality. However, perfectionism is an unfair and unrealistic demand. Have you, or someone you know done an amazing job…except for…one small (or large) mistake? We have all been there.

  What is so fascinating is that people often fixate on the one isolated mistake, rather than seeing it within the context of the larger task. While you should not be cavalier about making mistakes, or take your work responsibilities lightly, it is okay to be human. Making mistakes does not make you a bad person – or bad employee. It simply means you are continuing to grow in your skills, knowledge and attributes.

  I encourage individuals to accept their current skill level, while working at increasing their skills with self-compassion and patience.

Chapter 3

Ergonomics and Overuse

There are essentially six high-risk ergonomic factors that people with overuse symptoms often employ. In many ways this is very good news. Personal work ergonomics are something over which each person can have a significant amount of control. It may take focus, awareness and a plan to develop healthier ergonomic behaviors – but it can be done. I have seen hundreds of people over the years do exactly that.

I do want to mention here that I am not suggesting you must have perfect ergonomics in every situation, at all times in order to avoid or manage an overuse injury. There are moments when each of us will exhibit less than perfect posture, or move in ways that are not completely graceful. *However, it is when high-risk ergonomic behaviors become the overriding style of work that it is problematic.*

In order to begin to remediate any high-risk ergonomic factors it is vital to:

1) Be aware of what these risk factors are,

2) Determine whether or not you are engaging in any risk factors,

3) Replace the high risk factor with a lower risk strategy.

All three of these steps are essential in order to reduce the risk of injury. While this may seem straightforward, it is not always quite so easy to do alone.

It seems to be very difficult for people to identify their own personal high risk ergonomics without help and without training. It's like trying to diagnose your own symptoms of disease using the Internet. My suggestion is to seek assistance from someone who can help you in pinpointing your ergonomic strengths and weaknesses.

The ergonomic factors to be explored are:

- ♣ Appropriate use of force

- ♣ Healthy use of work-space

- ♣ Micro rest-breaks

- ♣ Hand/wrist positioning

- ♣ Physical muscle tension
- ♣ Posture

Force:

It is essential to modulate the force used when working or playing. Research has demonstrated that the greater the force utilized when performing a task, the greater the risk of overuse injury. For example, many people type with a lot of force on the keyboard with their fingers, or run with a significant impact force when their foot hits the ground. Both of these examples place the person at risk for injury. When I conduct ergonomic assessments, it is probably one of the risk factors I see most often. This style of ergonomics or body mechanics is often called "ballistic".

It is typified by:

- ♣ Movements with quick, abrupt starts (acceleration) and stops;
- ♣ Contact force which may, or may not, elicit sound;
- ♣ "Bouncing" quality to movement;
- ♣ Extraneous movement of the whole body due to force.

One of the challenges I present to people who utilize a lot of force in their work and movements is to consider the questions:

- ♣ "How little force is required to do this task?" Or,
- ♣ "If you weren't allowed to use any force at all to do the task, how would you do it?"

This encourages the exploration and incorporation of other approaches as opposed to using force as a consistent default.

Workspace:

Your work-space can be too large or too small. There are unique challenges when either style is consistently utilized. If the space you use to do your work or activity is too large, the muscles can become fatigued very quickly. The further away from the body the arms are held, especially for extended periods of time, the greater the risk of injury.

Consider this: If I hold a glass of water at arm's length, my muscles will tire much more quickly than if I hold the glass closer to my body. This is because the muscles are working much harder the further my arms are held from my body. It stands to reason that a consistently large work-space can significantly increase the risk of getting an overuse injury.

Likewise, an extremely small work-space can contribute to a variety of unhealthy ergonomic consequences. When a task is performed too close to the body, or in a very confined space, mobility of the upper arm is reduced. As a result, the wrists, and sometimes the elbows, become hyper-mobile in order to compensate. This can lead to elbow and/or wrist pain.

A work space that is too small or too close to the body may also cause the shoulders to become hunched as the body attempts to adjust to the arm position. This can lead to an imbalance of the muscles in the upper back, shoulders and neck, resulting in fatigue and overuse symptoms.

When one's workspace is too high, it requires a tremendous amount of physical exertion to maintain the arm in the air. This can contribute to muscle spasms and straining of the wrist and elbow joints as they try to absorb the workload. This can result in micro-tears of soft tissue that over time can become cumulative.

Though there are many exceptions, a healthy workspace in which a variety of tasks may generally be performed safely is:

* **Height** = about waist level to the chest

* **Width** = about shoulder width.

* **Depth** = extends to about three fourths of the fully extended arm.

Note: *The workspace employed may vary depending on the task involved.* For example you wouldn't want to use a keyboard that was chest level. Likewise, you wouldn't want to bowl keeping your hands at the level of the waist or above! Each task should be assessed individually to determine the healthiest workspace for that particular endeavor. Generally one should move within the determined workspace in a natural way as opposed to only within one quadrant or part of the space.

Micro rest breaks:

Micro rest breaks are different than rest and recovery time. Rest and recovery time refers to "down time" *between* times of activity, affording your body time to recoup from exertion. Micro rest breaks are those moments when you put one or both hands onto your lap if sitting, and to your side if standing - *while you are working.*

Research conducted by OSHA shows that when the hand(s) is placed onto the lap, *even for microseconds* while working, it significantly reduces post-work symptoms of fatigue and pain. A question I am frequently asked by people is, "But doesn't it take a lot more work to put the hands down for a micro-second, only to have to bring them *all the way back up* right away?" While that may *seem* to make sense, consider whether it is more fatiguing to hold a two pound weight out in front of you for 30 minutes straight, or to intersperse it with brief moments when your hand and arms are lowered.

I have observed many people folding their hands and "resting" them on their chest or abdomen. These are not true rests. While they are certainly better than leaving the arms up, they are not as effective as lowering the hands into the lap for a full rest.

Hand/wrist positioning:

While some movements may require a deviation, or bending, of the hand and wrist area, the position of the hand and wrist should remain in neutral position as much as is possible. Neutral position means that the hand, wrist and forearm are in alignment.

According to OSHA, hand/wrist deviations from neutral position are associated with greater pain and fatigue following work. An increase in the number of hand/wrist deviations from neutral position significantly increases the risk for overuse injury.

There may be a number of underlying root causes for excessive hand/wrist deviations:

♣ Failure to rest the non-dominant hand when it is not being used during a task can be problematic. If the hand is left hanging in the air it will often sag – which is a deviation from the neutral position of the hand/wrist.

- Working too close to the body can encourage improper hand and wrist positioning. If the arms are too close to the body during an activity or work task, this can create a hypo-mobility of the upper arm and a hyper-mobility of the wrist. When the wrist becomes hyper-mobile it results in a hand/wrist deviation.

- Working in an excessively high work space will often directly lead to hand/wrist deviations. Try holding your hands near your face with your palms facing each other. Now, while keeping that hand position point straight ahead. Notice your wrist is slightly bent. Now, while keeping your hands in the same position, lower your hands and notice what happens. Simply lowering the arm and hand often eliminates the hand/wrist deviation.

- Development of an overly "relaxed" style or work or play can cause hand/wrist deviations. While being relaxed during work and play is important, there does need to be a measured amount of control over the movement of the body.

- Sometimes there is a lack of knowledge or awareness of how to perform an activity or work without a hand/wrist deviation. In this case it may be helpful to have an ergonomic expert or an occupational therapist do an assessment and help you identify new and healthier approaches.

Physical muscle tension:

If you are physically tense, then you are more susceptible to an overuse injury. This is true for several reasons. First, since tense muscles are less flexible, the risk for micro-tears increases. This is especially true if there are concurrent forceful movements or excessive hand/wrist deviations.

Increased muscle tension may also adversely affect the circulation of blood to the extremities. Adequate blood supply to the extremities is needed to perform any work or activity safely. Blood carries needed oxygen to the cells to vitalize the muscles and soft tissue. Additionally, ample blood supply is essential to repair soft tissue that has been taxed during exertion. It is vital that you approach your work or sport in a relaxed and comfortable style. As mentioned in the previous chapter, some of the causes of physical muscle tension include:

♣ Emotional tension.

♣ Learned muscle patterns.

♣ Static Loading (holding muscles in a "static" position long enough to create physical muscle tension)

Posture:

It is important to feel comfortable and relaxed while working, playing, sitting, or performing any task. A proper posture can contribute to this end. From an Oriental medical perspective, healthy posture is very important. It allows the energy of the body to flow unimpeded. Poor posture may cause an interruption in the flow of energy - much like a kink in a water hose can interrupt the flow of water. There is a famous saying in Oriental medicine that states "There is no pain if there is free flow; if there is pain, there is no free flow." So it is important to develop proper posture in order to decrease the risk of pain. Some specific benefits of a healthy posture include:

- Aligns bones and joints so that muscle movement is balanced.
- Helps decrease wear and tear on joint, thereby reducing the risk of arthritis.
- Decreases the stress on the ligaments.
- Promotes muscles balance on both sides of the spine, reducing pain and symptoms from muscle spasms, vertebral subluxations, and scoliosis.
- Increases overall energy since:
  - Qi (vital energy of the body) is flowing unimpeded.
  - Muscle contractions and tension are not draining energy from the body.
- Improves appearance.

Many of us have unconsciously developed unhealthy posture. This can be a result of several contributing factors including:

- Engaging in body habits or exercises that overuse or strengthen certain muscle groups, while leaving other muscle groups underdeveloped. (For example, the abdominal muscles may be too weak to help support the proper low back position, or the hamstring muscles may be too tight, causing the pelvis to rotate backwards. This produces an abnormal slouching posture.)

- Compensatory postural adjustments due to trauma or injury.
- Suppression of feelings and emotions that, left unprocessed, manifest in our posture. This can easily be demonstrated by observing the posture of someone who is excited and happy compared to someone who is depressed and sad. Having said that, consciously choosing and practicing proper posture as a point of intervention can actually help balance the body and emotions (to demonstrate this point, try feeling sad for any length of time with a great posture!).

But what *is* proper posture? And how do you go about developing it? And, does having proper posture mean you have to sit or stand like an uncomfortable automaton all the time?

A healthy posture requires that the entire back and neck be properly aligned. The neck, or cervical spine, should curve slightly inward. The mid back, or thoracic spine, curves outward. And the low back, or lumbar spine, should curve inward. If any of these curvatures is lacking, then the posture of the entire body is compromised.

Focusing on the position of the head when attempting to achieve healthy posture can be helpful. The body seems to naturally follow where the head leads. If the head is stooped or juts forward, the rest of the body will 'slump.' If the head is erect and properly aligned, the rest of the body will most likely be as well. A generally healthy posture can be described as follows:

- Sitting:

  o Feet flat on the floor.
  o Thighs parallel to the floor.
  o Knees even with, or slightly higher than the hips.
  o Back straight and shoulders comfortably back.
  o Buttocks lightly touching the back of the chair.

- o   Normal curvature of the back.
- o   Both buttocks square on the chair, with weight distributed evenly.
- o   Legs ideally uncrossed; if legs are crossed, keep hips aligned on the chair and alternate the crossed legs.
- o   Change positions often to avoid static loading of muscles.

- • Standing:

  - o   Both feet flat on the floor
  - o   Weight distributed evenly across foot
  - o   Knees flexible, not locked
  - o   Head held up
  - o   Shoulder blades back and yet relaxed
  - o   Chin slightly tucked
  - o   Knees directly over ankles
  - o   Hips directly over knees
  - o   Stomach slightly tucked into enhance natural curvature of the lower back
  - o   Shoulders directly over hips
  - o   Ears directly over shoulders
  - o   The top of the head feels like it is being pulled upward.

- • Sleeping:

  - o   A position which helps maintain the curve in your back.
  - o   Avoid sleeping on stomach, especially on a soft mattress.
  - o   A pillow under the knees if sleeping on back.
  - o   A pillow between the knees if sleeping on side.
  - o   Alternate sides if sleeping on your side.

It is important to not confuse a healthy posture with a stiff and rigid positioning of the body. I like to think of healthy posture as our 'default' position – a centered and aligned stance from which we move and function. Body movements and postures should be fluid, relaxed and integrated. Changing positions every so often is a great way to allow your body to remain stress free and supple.

A balanced, natural and healthy posture ensures optimal muscle function. An imbalance can cause excessive wear and tear, which can eventually lead to pain and chronic symptoms. It is my observation that one of the most common reasons for neck and shoulder pain is poor posture. It is worth the time and energy to develop a healthy posture.

Chapter 4

Developing Low Risk Ergonomics

Developing low risk ergonomics is essential to the prevention and management of overuse injury. It is, of course, not sufficient to simply identify the high risk ergonomics in which you may engage. The high risk ergonomic behaviors must be replaced with lower risk ones in order to be effective. This chapter provides some general strategies that you can apply to your specific activity or work.

General Strategies for Your Consideration

- **Set aside at least 10 minutes a day to practice healthy ergonomics.** When developing any skill it is important to establish a regular time for practice. Developing low risk ergonomics is no exception. Just ten minutes a day can make a substantial difference in the quality and health of your ergonomics.

- **Find a model to observe, learn from and emulate.** It can be helpful to find someone who demonstrates low risk ergonomics in areas you are attempting to remediate. You can learn a great deal observing the various low risk ways in which they move and work.

- **Use visualization techniques to imagine yourself working in a low risk fashion.** This can be especially helpful to people who are currently dealing with an injury and are concerned that extra practice time could exacerbate their symptoms. Visualization has proven to be extremely effective in the development and refinement of a wide variety of skills and can be employed to develop low risk ergonomics. The brain simply does not know the difference between what is real and what is imagined. This is why you can awaken from a bad dream with your heart pounding and dripping wet from sweat, or can feel a twinge of anxiety if you simply close your eyes and imagine a tarantula getting ready to crawl up your leg. Visualization can be utilized for the purpose of building healthier ergonomics.

- **Eliminate high-risk ergonomic behaviors one at a time.** Select one or two fairly common high risk ergonomic behaviors that you intend to remediate immediately. For example, you may decide to keyboard without excessive hand/wrist deviations from now on - no matter what. Once you have fully incorporated that change into your work style, you can target one or two more ergonomic risk factors for remediation. In this way you begin to systematically shift your high risk ergonomic ways of moving to those of a lower risk style.

- **Have an ergonomic expert observe your work and provide feedback**. This can be a helpful ongoing strategy. You receive feedback on your progress as you work to make changes.

- **During *practice time* strive for the "extreme opposite" of the behavior you are trying to remedy.** For example, if you are seeking to develop a less forceful work style, then strive for an extremely "soft" style during practice time. If you are focusing on learning to work with less tension, pretend your limbs are like wet noodles, etc. This doesn't mean you will be doing your *work or activity* in this extreme fashion, but that you will garner the benefit of experiencing what "non-force" feels like, or what complete relaxation is like, and so on, when practicing.

- **Commit to learn *and use* at least one new way of moving differently every week.** Look for opportunities to incorporate what you learn into your work during the course of the day so that it becomes a part of you. This can be a great way to add a little creativity into your work. It can be fun to see how many times you can utilize a new skill. Of course it must be appropriate to the setting or it should not be utilized. The goal is for the newly learned skill to augment your current skills, not to skew it just because you want to "try out" something new.

- **Focus on changing your ergonomics during practice time, and slowly begin to incorporate these changes into your work or activity.** Attempting substantial ergonomic changes during your actual work, sport, or other activity can result in a serious breakdown of your ability to perform any task at full peak. It may be more effective to *practice* these new strategies first.

- **Give yourself time and permission to make mistakes and to move slowly.** Changing habituated ergonomic patterns is not a quick fix.

It takes time and awareness. You *will* make mistakes. Beating yourself up for mistakes will slow your progress.

♣ **Relax and have fun.** This may be a challenge if you don't enjoy what you are doing. Of course, that can contribute to the risk of injury too. At least make sure that you are including time for fun and relaxation into your life. This promotes the flow of a variety of "feel good" chemicals in your body that promotes healing.

Strategies for Healthy Force

♣ **During practice time, move or work to the rhythm of music.** Go with the flow and try to move as "softly" as possible. This will support a rhythm and flow to your movements (as long as it is not acid rock!).

♣ **Visualize yourself moving underwater during practice time.** This helps to create a sensation of complete relaxation and buoyancy in your movements. It can help to reduce the force and speed with which you move through space.

♣ **Videotape your work or activity and LISTEN to it.** Force is often, though not always, accompanied by sound. If you can hear yourself then you may be moving or working too forcefully.

Strategies for Healthy Posture

♣ **Sit on a "no-slip" pad.** Sometimes people begin their workday with proper posture, only to start what I call the "slow slide." Within a few minutes their rear ends are hugging the edge of the chair and their backs are more horizontal to the seat of the chair than perpendicular. A no-slip pad, purchased in any department store, is a quick remedy.

♣ **Keep both feet on the floor.** This is ideal. However most people prefer to cross their legs. If that is your style, I advice switching crossed legs frequently and keeping your hips square on the chair as opposed to leaning on one buttock.

♣ **Experiment with the "feel" of proper posture.** A healthy posture can take a while to get used to; however, it can make a significant difference in your body's ability to sustain long periods of sitting or standing.

♣ **Practice optimum posture during your leisure time.** You cannot have poor posture in every other area of your life and expect to maintain a healthy stance while working or engaged in your sport! It is important to foster good posture when you are not engaged in anything specific so that it becomes your natural default position.

♣ **Be aware of your head position.** Where your head goes, your body will follow. If your head is in alignment, your body will most likely follow suit.

Strategies for Healthy Hand/Wrist Positions

♣ **Incorporate more muscle groups into work.** I often see people use as few muscles groups as possible when they work - in an effort to protect their arms. This can be counter-productive. In reality the more muscle groups that are employed, the less the risk of injury. This can be easily demonstrated by observing someone attempting to move a 200 pound stone. If he or she tries to do it alone it can be very difficult. However, with the help of two or three additional people the load becomes light. Ensuring the mobility and cooperation of all pertinent muscle groups helps to minimize overtaxing one muscle group.

♣ **Experiment with the orientation and height of your hand, palm and fingers when moving and working.** This can affect whether a movement is produced with low or high risk ergonomics. For example, the height of your hands can affect whether or not a hand/wrist deviation from neutral positioning takes place. A simple adjustment of height can sometimes eliminate this high risk work style.

♣ **Incorporate more rest breaks when your non-dominant hand is not in use.** The non-dominant hand inevitably will sag and result in a hand/wrist deviation if allowed to hang in mid-air while not in use. Lowering the non-dominant hand onto the lap when it is not in use not only prevents deviations from neutral wrist positioning, but also provides momentary relief to the shoulder muscles.

- ♣ **Relax!** If your forearm muscles are tense this could cause a resulting hyper-mobility in the hand/wrist area. When one area of your body is less mobile, other parts of the body must become hyper-mobile to compensate. If the forearm muscles are tense, there is a reduction in movement of the forearm, resulting in hyper-mobility of the hand and wrist.

- ♣ **Place a mirror in your work or practice space.** Observe yourself as you work and practice your skills. It is challenging to notice or feel your own hand/wrist deviations. Observing yourself in a mirror or even on videotape can help you see deviations that you might not otherwise notice.

- ♣ **Place tape on the back of your hand and wrist area during practice.** This can increase awareness of times when you are working with hand/wrist deviations.

- ♣ **Make sure your work-space is not too close to the body**. Sometimes people work close to the body in an attempt to protect sore upper arm or shoulders. However, this can create additional overuse symptoms over time. When the work-space is too close to the body, the upper arms and forearms become less mobile resulting in hyper-mobility of the hand/wrist area.

Strategies for Reducing Tension

- ♣ **Take deep breaths often.** In the chapter addressing stress management I detail the many benefits of breathing. One of the payoffs is a significant reduction in both mental and physical tension. There are many missed opportunities to breathe. In Oriental medicine it is said that 'The life is in the breath!"

- ♣ **LOWER your shoulders.** When combined with breathing, lowering the shoulders can make a huge difference in the levels of pain and fatigue. Many people can easily and quickly lower their shoulders with a moment of awareness. What is interesting is that if you can lower you shoulders, then you are tense, otherwise your shoulders would not have been elevated. Many people carry much more tension than they are aware of. Using this simple exercise can help bring awareness and help you to release tension.

- **While maintaining proper posture, purposefully get in a very relaxed physical position.** If your body is relaxed, your mind will follow. The mind-body connection is powerful. It is not possible to be physically tense, while at the same time mentally relaxed. Likewise you can't be mentally tense and physically relaxed. If you find yourself feeling tension, then a simple remedy is to relax and release your muscles. There is a quick method called "progressive relaxation" that is very effective. Begin by relaxing your feet muscles and work up your body. As you notice a tense muscle or muscle group simply mentally release them. As you do so, not only will your physical tension lessen, but so too will your mental stress.

- **Practice relaxing at least 10 minutes daily.** The benefits of doing so are well documented. Sometimes life is busy and filled with noisy distraction. It is easy to habituate a state of stress and tension. Relaxing for even a few minutes a day can help bring you back to a state of awareness and calmness. I personally meditate for one hour each morning before starting my day. I am then able to make decisions and perform my daily tasks from a calm center.

- **Limit caffeine prior to work or physical activities.** Caffeine is a stimulant and can create substantial tension when used in excess. Prior to repetitive work may not be the best time to consume substances that increase tension.

- **Eat foods that nourish your nervous system.** The importance of a healthy diet cannot be overstated. It absolutely affects your risk of overuse in a variety of ways, only one of which is to provide the nervous system with what it needs in order to maintain a sense of composure and calmness.

Strategies for a Healthy Work Space

- **Put a mirror in your work space in order to monitor your use of work space.** This will enable you to observe how effectively you utilize your space.

- **Clear away clutter.** This will enable your to move freely in space without obstacles.

- ♣ **Create a healthy ergonomic work station.** Tips on how to do this can be found in chapter 12.

- ♣ **Make sure the tools you most often use in your work are within easy grasp.** Stress on the upper extremity increases with repeated reaches for objects that are far away. This can contribute to overuse injury and exacerbate current symptoms.

Strategies for Incorporating Rest Time During Work

- ♣ **Have someone count your one-handed and two-handed rest breaks during your practice time.** It is amazing to see how these small micro-second rests can be utilized.

    As I mentioned before, people often ask me, "Isn't it more work to put the hand down and then have to bring it all the way back up again?" At first blush that may seem logical. However, consider the muscle fatigue you would most likely experience if you held your arm straight in front of you without rest for an hour compared to that you might experience if you periodically put your hand down – even if just for a moment.

    When one or both hands are lowered, there is a corresponding relief to all of the adjacent muscle groups. Additionally, putting your hands down - even for a second or two - minimizes "static loading" of the muscles. Static loading occurs when muscles are not allowed relief, and the results are tension and spasms.

- ♣ **Post reminders to yourself in your environment to rest.** I have seen people work for as much as an hour or more without putting their hands down once. When this pattern of work has been habituated it can take time and focus to initiate change. Sometimes visual cues can be helpful as you begin to increase your awareness and choose healthier ergonomic behaviors. They can be a helpful reminder to take the time to rest.

Chapter 5

Rest and Recovery Time

In addition to incorporating micro-rest breaks, appropriate rest and recovery time is an important aspect for the prevention of overuse injury. If the body is not being given sufficient recovery time, the risk of injury increases. Your body needs time to rest. Overuse injury generally occurs as a result of multiple micro injuries. Your body needs time to repair and heal itself. Pacing yourself and building in adequate time to heal should be a primary professional and personal consideration. Each person has different needs, but some helpful guidelines are:

♣ **Ensure that you are interspersing heavier and lighter tasks**. This guarantees greater balance in your work life and schedule. Certainly there may be times when a special "high demand" task or activity may arise. However such situations should be extraordinary. Exceptions do happen, but you must take care to ensure that the exceptions do not become common practice as you frame your schedule and life. Each endeavor should be considered within the larger scope of the "heavier followed by lighter" principle. This helps ensure a life that is balanced and manageable.

♣ **Advocate for your needs.** This can feel "sticky" for some. One of the most common things people say to me is that their employers will not accommodate their needs. I have spoken with individuals who have had three carpal tunnel surgeries because the organization for which they worked would not "allow" them to have reasonable breaks or work with them to determine ways in which to accommodate their physical needs. While I do not advocate approaching things with an adversarial attitude, I also do not advocate laying your body on the altar of your job to avoid conflict.

I encourage you to place your needs first and foremost in all situations. This is **not** selfish! You are not doing anyone a favor if you create a disability. Then you will not be able to work or engage in some of your favorite activities *at all!* It is never healthy to present yourself as a martyr. And if the work demands are truly unsafe there are legal steps that may be taken to address them. The Occupational Health Administration (OSHA) can be contacted to conduct investigations into workplace safety practices.

♣ **Don't leave pain unaddressed.** If you are hurting, sore or feeling achy, your body is sending you a signal that you need rest and recovery time. Continuing to engage in the activity that caused the initial symptoms will only exacerbate the symptoms! It's like running with a sprained ankle. Everyone knows that running with a sprained ankle is a bad idea. It needs rest in order to heal. If you continue running while it is injured, the ankle will likely get worse. The same is true with issues regarding your upper extremities. Allowing your body to recuperate is one of the most powerful things you can do to reduce the risk of, and/or manage an existing overuse injury.

Chapter 6

Exercise to Increase Strength and Endurance

This chapter includes a variety of aspects, including warming up and cooling down prior to and following work and exertion of any kind, as well as increasing physical strength and endurance.

I do not intend to delineate specific strength and endurance exercises because there are a number of wonderful programs already available that can be utilized. It can be helpful to work with a physical therapist to develop a program appropriate for you if you are currently dealing with overuse symptoms.

In this chapter I plan to outline some basic principles that are important to keep in mind when considering developing an exercise program. I do strongly recommend that *everyone* make getting and keeping fit a high priority.

It is essential to develop the necessary strength and endurance for any task that taxes the body and presents the risk of overuse injury. The risk of injury significantly increases when muscles are not strong enough to handle a given task. Many sports, as well as work requiring repetitive motions, require a great deal of stamina. One of the easiest ways to *decrease* the injury risk is to *increase* physical strength.

It is very important to check with your health care provider prior to engaging in any exercise program.

Stretching

One aspect of exercise to address is that of stretching. I am not a proponent of the most common approach to stretching in America today. It generally involves stretching the muscle to the utmost (or very nearly) for a few seconds to a few minutes. I have treated many patients who have tried to increase their range of motion and flexibility utilizing this approach. This way of stretching can often result in or exacerbate an injury. I encourage my patients to try is a softer approach to stretching.

Muscles that could benefit from some lengthening are tight and tense, which is why they need to be stretched. The problem is that people stretch muscles like rubber bands. When you stretch a rubber band it gets tight and it also weakens! So I believe that to stretch a "tight" muscle in a "tight" way leads to a muscle memory of tightness. It also has the potential to weaken the muscle.

Sometimes there is a shortening of the muscle fibers in response to stretching techniques that are too aggressive. This is the body's efforts to protect a muscle it perceives as being over stretched. The muscles "feel" attacked when stretched in this way.

I have seen *dramatically* positive results with a much softer approach. For example, I had a patient who was training for a marathon. This individual had run many marathons in the past, but this time found himself running with an 8 out of 10 pain level during training (0 = no pain, 10 = the worse pain possible). He had been trying to stretch his hamstrings in the typical fashion; however, things were simply getting worse after 4 months. He had been receiving acupuncture from another practitioner and decided to come to see me at the recommendation of a friend.

In addition to acupuncture treatments, I suggested he try a different approach to stretching that I call "moving into softness." The stretching movements are the same as usual, but performed with a different intensity and focus. Instead of trying to move the muscles into the biggest stretch possible, I suggested that if it "felt" like a stretch he was *going too far!* I explained that if he made sure he did not stretch beyond the point that he could *completely* relax his hamstring muscle, then his muscle would actually begin to "let go" and lengthen. I told him that he could move a little further into the stretch once his muscles got used to that position, as long as he was still able to keep his hamstring perfectly relaxed in the new position as well. Within 1 week he was running with 50% less pain, and within three weeks he was running without pain.

Often, with a little time, people are able to stretch even further than when they were "cranking" the stretch – and without the negative rebound effect of the body trying to guard and protect itself from the aggressive stretch. It just takes a little more time. This approach teaches the muscles to be stretched AND relaxed!

Warming Up and Cooling Down

Warming up and cooling down prior to and following exertion is a significant part of professional and personal self-care.

The same exercises can be done for both warming up and cooling down. Let's look at the function of warming up and cooling down separately:

Warming Up

Gentle warming-up of the entire body is optimal. Warming up helps prepare the muscles, tendons, ligaments and blood vessels for activity. It increases flexibility and circulation to the entire body, including the upper extremities. This greatly reduces the risk of overuse injury.

Caution with Warming Up: Warm up movements should be measured and performed with *control.* This is extremely important, *especially if you are experiencing current overuse injury symptoms!* Uncontrolled movements and abrupt gesticulations such as shaking the hands, or ballistic, forceful movements do not allow the body time to adjust and can strain soft tissue and joints.

Systemic Warm Up: A systemic warm up can be as simple as a brisk walk or isometric exercises. The goal is the get your blood circulating, resulting in more efficient oxygenation of the whole body, including the extremities. If you try to warm up the extremities in isolation, without a total warm up, the effect is short lived and incomplete. Your body works as a whole unit. Sometimes I see people trying to warm up by running their hands under hot water. While this can certainly be helpful if you are coming in out of freezing temperatures, do not be fooled into thinking that it has made your muscles ready for work. It can help create a short term, localized effect, but if the circulation of the whole body is not stimulated, the circulation of blood to the hands and arms *will* be short lived.

Targeted Warm Up: After a systemic warm up, gentle movements may be done that mimic the task you will be performing. These movements will help gently warm the specific muscles involved. The goal is to increase the mobility and flexibility of the hands and arms so they are ready for the activity.

Cooling Down

Cooling down, though often ignored, is as important as the warm up. It allows the body to remove residue waste products produced during exertion, such as lactic acid. These waste products are by and large responsible for the soreness that results from exercise performed without the benefit of cooling down. Cooling down also allows the body to gently return to homeostasis. It helps to expedite the recovery process since residual waste products impede healing.

Chapter 7

Stress Management

Many people in the health care field now believe that stress plays a greater part in the risk of injury and disease than previously thought and can significantly impact the body's ability to heal. It affects brain function, the cardiovascular system, the nervous system, the endocrine system, and the digestive system (including the ability to assimilate nutrients from the foods eaten). All of this, of course, impacts the risk of overuse injury.

Feeling emotionally stressed is an experience we all share at one time or another. From an Oriental medical perspective emotional stress can certainly create imbalance in the body, which makes it susceptible to injury, illness and disease. The Neijing, the oldest and most authoritative Oriental medical text, says that overindulgence in emotions can create imbalances in the body.[8]

Unbalanced emotions can lead to impairment of Qi (pronounced Chee), Blood and Yin. Qi is essentially the body's energy system. If Qi does not flow freely, or is depleted or impaired in some way, emotions will be negatively affected. Blood is considered to be the physical basis for the Shen, or Spirit, which includes the emotional and mental aspect of your life. If there is disharmony with the Blood, there isn't the needed foundation for healthy, balanced emotions. Yin is essential to moisten and nourish your body and to "anchor" your more Yang, or dynamic energies.

Just as the harmony of Qi, Blood and Yin is necessary for emotional well-being, your physical health may be affected, either negatively or positively, by your emotions. Repressed or over-indulged emotions and stress, such as anger, mania, sadness or worry, can result in illness. In the same way, illness and disease may disrupt emotional balance. In order to reduce stress it can be helpful to maintain daily practices designed to reduce stressful thinking and increase a positive mindset.

From a Western perspective the experience of stress also has been demonstrated to impact your risk of overuse injury. It increases muscle tension, decreases blood flow to the extremities, increases the body's autonomic functions, decreases mental function and increases pain levels.

There are many effective methods for reducing the experience of stress in your life. It is not my intention to address each method in depth. I have addressed some of them with varying levels of depth below:

- **Acupuncture:** Acupuncture is an incredible modality for balancing the energies of the body, resulting in a reduction of stressful feelings. It has been shown to stimulate endorphins and other chemicals in the body that elevate mood, assist in healing and promote sound sleep.

- **Meditation.** There are many forms of meditation that can be helpful. Find the specific "style" that best suits your needs. The goal is to schedule time daily when you are able to quiet your mind and enter a state of calmness. Some people experience this as connecting with their "Higher Power," while other people simply see it as an opportunity to momentarily leave the business of life and sit quietly. Whatever it means for you is perfectly fine, but experts in the health field overwhelmingly agree that daily meditation can be an extremely helpful addition for those seeking to reduce stress.

- **Eat to feel good.** Your brain literally uses the food you eat as the raw material from which to make the chemicals it needs to help you feel good. Chapter 9 is dedicated to the topic of nutritional interventions to manage pain and to support emotional health.

- **Practice a positive mindset.** It has been said that situations cannot cause stress, but feelings of stress are the result of stressful thinking. Many psychotherapists believe emotions are actually a result of thought. This means that thoughts give birth to emotions rather than the other way around. If you are feeling sad, the sadness was generated by a specific thought.

  The same would be true of all emotions, including feelings of anger, frustration, joy, excitement, etc. The idea is that if a situation can be stressful in and of itself, then everyone would experience stress if exposed to the very same situation. This is not usually the case. For example, one person who is given the task to write a speech for the mayor might feel extremely stressed, while someone else might be energized and exhilarated by the challenge.

  If thoughts truly do generate emotions, then it may be prudent to be aware of what your thoughts are, and to nurture those that encourage positive and empowered emotions.

♣ **Lower your tolerance _for_ stress.** At first blush this may seem a bit counter intuitive; however, it can help to greatly reduce your experience of stress. It is a matter of honoring the need for a balanced life, as well as having a keen sense of the stressors in your life. Often people try to power through situations, or just "suck it up" rather than focusing on initially setting healthy boundaries. If you feel too busy and overwhelmed in your daily life, you may be tolerating and accepting too much stress into your life.

It is important to recognize and address potential stressors. Of course we all need to develop internal fortitude and strength in the face of adversity. However, that is very different than allowing the fodder for stress to muddy your life. Consider, for example, how much frustration you might experience while working if you accepted a job for which you truly did not have the skills to perform. You most probably would experience feelings of stress - the same stress could be prevented by simply turning down the assignment. It is making a conscious choice to not accommodate avoidable stressors in your life.

Lowering your tolerance for stress is a pro-active approach to experiencing more peace and balance in your life. Placing a high premium on living a balanced lifestyle will prompt you to take appropriate action when something threatens to compromise that balance.

♣ **Get adequate sleep.** Sleep is a vital ingredient for maintaining health and to enhance healing. A substantial amount of healing actually takes place during deep sleep. Symptoms mimicking fibromyalgia and chronic fatigue syndrome can be elicited by denying even a few nights worth of deep sleep. One reason for this is that human growth hormone peaks during deep sleep. Recent research has also shown that people who do not sleep enough tend to eat hundreds more calories per day than if they got adequate sleep. Because sleep difficulties have become such a scourge in American society, I often advise people to maintain what is commonly known as "sleep hygiene."

Good sleep hygiene contributes greatly to consistent and restful, healing sleep. Some aspects of sleep hygiene include:

○ Try to go to bed and get up at the same times every day. This allows your internal clock to "set." Your body will start to get tired as you approach bedtime when you develop a pattern.

- Try to schedule sleep times aligned with the natural rhythms of nature. This means being awake during the daylight hours and sleeping at night. In Oriental medicine getting in synch with the natural rhythms of the world is very important. It is 'going with the grain' rather than against it.

- Lighten up your morning with some sunshine. Light helps reduce levels of melatonin in the brain (the sleep hormone) and increases serotonin (which helps you feel good, but calm). This too will help to regulate your hormones for optimal sleep.

- Be careful of too much caffeine intake, especially in the afternoon and evening.

- Avoid alcohol within four or five hours prior to bedtime. While alcohol may help some people fall asleep faster, it tends to cause a delayed sleep disturbance.

- Avoid eating heavily in the evenings. It has been said that if you eat late at night you will either digest well or sleep well - but not both. Heavy, greasy and spicy foods are of particular concern.

- Do not do anything in bed other than sleep or sex since you want your brain to associate bed with sleep.

- Engage in calming activities prior to bed. Relaxation techniques such as deep breathing can help the body decompress from the day. Television and computer work can actually stimulate the brain.

- Avoid vigorous exercise within two hours of going to bed.

- If you have trouble "turning off your mind," try soaking just your feet in very warm water for 15 minutes prior to bed. In Ohinese medicine this is believed to bring the energy down and out of the head. I have seen this make a real difference for people.

- Make sure your sleeping environment is comfortable, quiet, dark and at a moderate temperature.

- Establish a ritual prior to bedtime. This sends your brain a signal to also prepare for sleep.

- If you do not fall asleep within a half hour, get out of bed and read a book (not a white knuckle thriller…) until you feel sleepy, then go back to bed.

- Do not try to go to sleep. Allow yourself to "daydream." Going to sleep is a natural process. Trying to fall asleep actually will cause tension that prevents the natural process.

♣ **Breathe:** Breathing is, of course, vital to life! It supplies your body with oxygen, and it also helps eliminate toxins and metabolic waste products, including accumulated carbon dioxide. Literally *every cell* in the body needs sufficient oxygen to function healthily. This is important because *decreased* levels of oxygen contribute greatly to fatigue and inhibit the natural ability of the body to heal from injury and disease. Some benefits of deep breathing that directly reduce the risk of overuse injury include:

- It is essential for healthy brain function. This greatly affects your ability to process information in a clear and helpful way while working.

- It enhances your body's ability to recover and heal from injury and disease.

- It helps your body eliminate toxins.

- It assists in the digestion of food and assimilation of nutrients from the foods you eat.

- It oxygenates the nervous system, which interfaces with every system of your body.

- It provides oxygen to the glandular and hormonal systems. This is important because some hormonal problems can increase the risk of overuse injury.

o It affects the parasympathetic nervous system, resulting in more physical muscle relaxation. This can directly reduce the risk of overuse injury.

o It reduces anxiety, which is a risk factor for overuse injury.

♣ **Movement Therapies:** There are many movement therapies that can assist in the reduction of stressful feelings. Four of my favorites are:

o **Yoga:** Yoga, as a method, is famous for reducing stress, as well as stretching and relaxing the body. I believe it can be a helpful modality if approached with care and wisdom. I have been practicing yoga for more than 25 years and have noticed that sometimes people can get overly ambitious and hurt themselves with stretches and stances for which they are ill prepared. If you choose to do yoga, I encourage you to find an experienced, caring, licensed yoga instructor for instruction.

o **Feldenkrais Method:** Feldenkrais is great for anybody desiring to learn how to move in more integrated and healthy ways! It helps you learn to move with more ease and freedom, to carry less physical stress, and to recognize and stop moving in ways that cause pain. It utilizes gentle movement and focused awareness of the body and its movement as a medium to improve physical function, enhance fluidity and ease of movement, along with an increased range of motion. I have also seen it dramatically reduce pain and tension resulting from imbalanced and overly stressed muscles.

   The Feldenkrais Method utilizes principles of physics and proper ergonomic biomechanics in its carefully prescribed movements. These movements are intended to bring your attention to the areas of your body that are unbalanced due to lack of awareness. As you move through the sequence of movements, you learn new ways of moving and actually begin to exchange old neuromuscular patterns for new healthier ones. I typically recommend Moshe Feldenkrais' book entitled *Awareness through Movement* for people interested in learning more about The Feldenkrais Method.

o **Tai Chi:** Often called Tai Chi Chuan, this is an ancient form of self defense originating in China at least 2000 years ago. It is sometimes called "meditation in motion" due to the fact that it helps to connect the mind and body through its gentle, dance-like movements that are coordinated with the breath. I have noticed that this particular form of movement "therapy" is especially helpful for people coping with overuse issues because it helps teach ways to move the body through space softly, in alignment and with all parts of the body working together in harmony. Tai Chi, when practiced regularly, helps to significantly reduce stress, while increasing flexibility, energy, strength and coordination.

- **Qi Gong:** Qi Gong is a method designed to help balance and strengthen the Qi, or energy of the body, thereby assisting in the natural healing process. It is extremely powerful and effective.

Chapter 8

Pain Management

Preventing and/or managing pain is an important topic for people in professions or recreational activities that require repetitive motion. If there is inadequate rest and recovery time, the cumulative effects of the repetitive movements may put substantial strain on the muscles and tendons of the upper extremity. This can result in microscopic tears.

Additionally, tendons and their coverings, called sheaths, begin to rub together because of inadequate lubrication resulting from overuse. The tendons then become inflamed and irritated, resulting in pain, especially with movement. Along with managing the cumulative effects of repetitive motions on the body, some people may also cope with other chronic inflammatory conditions such as arthritis.

Pain management includes a wide scope of strategies that should be considered when dealing with an existing overuse injury. Certainly everything mentioned in this book has a place as part of a comprehensive pain management program. However, some modifications may be needed in order to accommodate an injury. For example, though the preventative strategies listed may be useful when employed in a pain management program, there is a caveat.

It is *absolutely vital* to determine if the extent or severity of your injury precludes your engaging in certain activities safely at all. You may need a break in order for your body to heal. If you *can* realistically continue to work with accommodations, it may be necessary to outline what those accommodations need to be. Some general things to consider when dealing with existing pain or injury include (note: some of these have already been discussed as part of a comprehensive prevention program, but deserve special mention here as well):

- **♣ Seek assistance from your health care practitioner regarding the status of your condition.** It is important to determine whether you can safely continue to work or if you need recovery time. Continually stressing an injured extremity can potentially lead to permanent consequences. It is no different than continuing to run on a sprained ankle. There is an appropriate time for everything, including time for healing and recovery.

- ♣ **Include prevention and management of overuse injury in your annual professional development goals.** Prevention and management is equally as important as developing technical skills in any field. It generally not only helps you perform the task more safely, but also often influences the skill being practiced in a positive way.

- ♣ **Deal with overuse injury symptoms immediately.** Too often people ignore initial symptoms in hopes that they will miraculously go away. In reality, if symptoms are not dealt with they will generally become worse. If, while injured, you approach your work or activity in the same manner that precipitated injury with a sustained injury, it will exacerbate the problem.

- ♣ **Balance extracurricular activities with your work.** Watch for hobbies that are of a repetitive nature. This does not mean that you cannot continue to do the things you love; it simply means you need to balance the various aspects of your life so that you can maintain your health.

- ♣ **Watch for high-risk ergonomic behavior in your everyday activities.** You can be sure that any high-risk ergonomics in your work or sport will show up in other areas of your life. If you keyboard forcefully, for example, then you probably do many things in your life in a forceful and ballistic manner. This would include such activities as writing, chopping food, etc.

- ♣ **Use stress reduction and pain management strategies.** Your experience of pain is strongly influenced by your levels of stress and perceptions of what the pain means for you. Stressful feelings affect your body in significant ways, including affecting your circulatory and endocrine, or hormonal systems. Additionally, the meaning you assign to your pain impacts the experience of pain. For example, my experience of pain will be different depending on whether I believe my stomach pain is due to cancer as opposed to the fact that I ate too much.

  Remember, stress also has some bearing on your ability to absorb nutrients. Chronic stress can result in stress hormones "hijacking" nutrient receptors on the cells. This can, of course, impact the body's ability to repair and heal.

♣ **Soak in Epsom Salt.** Soaking in magnesium sulfate crystals, commonly known as Epsom Salt, can assist with pain management. Magnesium sulfate is absorbed easily through pores of the skin and can benefit your body in a variety of ways. Magnesium is essential for the maintenance of appropriate calcium levels in the blood.

    Magnesium is necessary for the conduction of electrical impulses in the body, directly impacting the function of every cell and bodily system. Magnesium is also well known as the "relaxation mineral." It is a natural stress reliever - both physically and emotionally. Additionally, Epsom Salt has the capacity to remove toxins from your body, including heavy metals, via reverse osmosis. The result can be a reduction in muscle pain and inflammation.

    Epsom Salt also delivers sulfates (*not* sulfites) to your cells. Sulfates are more easily absorbed your skin than through the food you eat. Sulfates assist in forming brain tissue, joint proteins and the lining of the digestive tract. Sulfates have also been shown to help detoxify the body.

    The one important caution when using Epsom salts is that it can dry out the skin if overused. I generally recommend 2 cups in the bath, 1-2 times a week to start. This will enable you to gauge how your skin is going to react. This can be increased as needed and tolerated. If your skin starts to dry out, then reduce the amount, or take a break from using it for a while.

♣ **Use ice sparingly and with caution.** A question I am often asked by patients with chronic pain resulting from overuse is, "How often, and for how long, should I apply ice?" My answer often surprises people. I tell them, "I typically wouldn't ice an area of chronic pain!" Unfortunately, regular icing seems to have become standard practice as part of an ongoing "self-care" regimen for chronic pain, especially if it stems from an acute injury. While there may be some short term relief from nagging symptoms, this approach can have long term repercussions.

    While we are all familiar with the RICE approach to treating an acute injury - **R**est, **I**ce, **C**ompression, and **E**levation - I think this protocol has been mistakenly generalized to the treatment of chronic issues. There is a time and place for therapeutically icing an injury, however in Oriental medicine it is used sparingly and as a short term intervention. Even in Western medicine, the protocol for icing an acute injury is for the first 48-72 hours. From an Oriental medical perspective, *overuse* of ice, even for an acute injury, can exacerbate symptoms, and even *create* a chronic condition.

Swelling is often considered to be "bad" and that it should be eliminated. I wonder if this idea is a response to a cultural propensity to focus on symptoms, rather than the cause of symptoms. Swelling serves a purpose! The swelling mechanism is a very important aspect of the healing process. Swelling results from nutrient and enzyme rich fluids that bathe an injured area, assisting in the healing process and providing natural "splinting" for protection. The body is so wise! If these fluids are blocked, then the healing process is impeded and the injury is more likely to become a chronic problem.

This is not to say ice should never be used. Ice can be invaluable when used in a timely and targeted manner. Certainly it can help control pain immediately following a physical trauma, or help reduce severe swelling that is cutting off circulation. The problem arises when it is used too much or for too long.

From a Western medical approach, ice is thought to keep swelling and inflammation down, while heat is thought to increase inflammation. Oriental medicine teaches that ice decreases blood circulation as it reduces inflammation, while heat increases blood circulation. This is an important distinction. While the application of heat may not always be appropriate, especially if the area of concern is red or hot to the touch, it does not necessarily mean the application of ice is appropriate as an ongoing or daily treatment approach.

If the painful area is cold or stiff, then careful application of mild heat, for short periods of 15 minutes or less, may be useful to help increase the circulation of Qi and blood in the local area. This brings oxygen and needed nutrients to the injured site and flushes out acids that may have accumulated in the tissue. In this way warmth may actually assist in the reduction of swelling, as well as help prevent the development of scar tissue.

Oriental medicine tends to look to nature to learn about the internal workings of your body. In nature, ice slows things down; it hardens. Oriental medicine maintains that your body responds to ice much the same way. Ice slows the movement of fluids and Qi (energy), decreases blood circulation, and hardens tissue. In nature, movement is essential for life. Likewise the movement of Qi and blood through the injured area of the body is also vital.

When this flow is diminished or blocked, it can lead to "stagnant" Qi and blood. This is important from an Oriental medical perspective, because where there is stagnation, there is pain. Icing temporarily addresses the symptoms, while establishing the free flow of Qi and blood assists in the actual healing process.

So how does this apply to the person who may experience ongoing symptoms of chronic pain stemming from an injury? I stated that ice should typically be reserved for the first 24 – 48 hours of an acute injury. So when it comes to treating overuse symptoms, what is a working definition of "acute?"

Acute conditions tend to be severe and sudden in onset, while chronic conditions usually develop over time. However, it is possible to have an acute attack in the midst of a chronic syndrome, especially if there is an underlying "root" weakness in the body's energetic system, insufficient recovery time before resuming activities, or if poor ergonomics or other exacerbating factors are involved. This is the situation many face.

Even so, the continual application of ice can cause a stagnation of Qi and blood, thereby blocking the healing process. This can create and perpetuate a vicious cycle. It may be likened to someone taking Ibuprofen daily for headaches who begins to experience Ibuprofen induced "rebound" headaches. A cycle has been established which may be difficult to break.

The goal must be to address and remediate the root cause of the injury, not just symptoms of discomfort and swelling. As such, it is important to implement a multi-dimensional program designed to strengthen the body, as well as nourish and encourage the healthy flow of Qi and blood.

Acupuncture and Chinese herbs can be extremely important aspects of such a program. These modalities are designed to help harmonize and balance the flow of Qi and blood in the body. When Qi and blood are flowing freely, the body's natural healing process is engaged, and pain and swelling *naturally* decreases.

♣ **Eat to reduce inflammation and pain.** See Chapter 9 for details.

♣ **Use caution with braces.** Many people wear braces daily; sometimes for hours at a time. While there is a time and place for the judicious use of braces, I find that they are used in ways that often create long term difficulties. The problem with excessive use of braces is that joint mobility can diminish and the muscles may become dependent on the braces for support. This allows muscles to atrophy and grow weaker. This can create a challenge when these weaker muscles are called upon to sustain work.

I believe braces can be helpful for maintaining a neutral hand/wrist position during sleep, and when there is an acute situation requiring substantial stabilization of the area. However, I do not support long term use of braces while working. If you are unable to work safely without the use of a brace, taking some time off in order to recover might be helpful.

Chapter 9

A Plateful of Pain - or Energy?

Food is intended to give pleasure, as well as nourish, strengthen and energize your body. The problem is that most of us developed eating patterns that, while satisfying taste buds, do not optimally nourish. Certain foods increase the inflammatory response and pain levels in the body.

Eating pseudo-food filled with numerous chemicals has become commonplace. Many Americans can go for weeks without so much as eating a fresh green vegetable. The problem with this pattern for people dealing with overuse is that your body needs adequate nutrition in order to heal the myriad "micro traumas" and reduce the inflammation that can occur with overuse injury.

It is important to minimize foods that increase the body's inflammatory response and pain levels. Some commonly eaten foods and food additives have been shown in research studies to provoke an inflammatory response, cause cellular death and increase pain levels in the body.[9]

Avoiding foods and food additives known to increase pain and inflammation in the body, while concurrently adding foods and herbs that reduce inflammation can be an important part of a comprehensive program of preventing and managing pain. Eating foods that are natural and unprocessed is one of the easiest ways to ensure the foods you eat are nutritious and nourishing.

Some helpful things to know about diet and managing pain are:

♣ **Excitotoxins:** Monosodium glutamate (MSG), aspartame, yeast extract, textured protein and soy protein isolate (a common ingredient in many soy-based meat substitute products) and refined sugars are among the culprits that may be implicated in the increase of pain levels in the body. These substances are considered to be "excitotoxins."

Excitotoxins are toxins known to hyper-stimulate and excite neurons, the primary cells of the nervous system. This can lead to injury, or even death, of the neurons. Additionally, these foods can cause the body to release several neuropeptides, or amino acids, two of which are "Substance P" and glutamate. Substance P is an important link in the transmission of pain signals in the body. It can also increase the body's inflammatory response that is intricately associated with pain. Glutamate functions directly as an excitotoxin.

Eating excitotoxic foods not only can increase and sharpen a person's experience of pain, but has also been shown to negatively impact a number of neurological and other disorders including fibromyalgia, migraine headaches, various skin diseases, and seizures, as well as some autoimmune disorders.

- ♣ **Food and the Inflammatory response:**
    - ○ **Don't:**
        - ▪ Eat too much animal protein. It contains arachidonic acid which can contribute to inflammation and pain if eaten in excess. It is commonly found in meat, eggs, and shellfish.

        - ▪ Eat too much sugar or refined products due to their inflammatory producing quality.

    - ○ **Do:**
        - • Take Fish Oil (unless you are allergic to fish, have a food sensitivity to fish or are on a blood thinner). Fish oil is one of the things I prescribe most to patients dealing with issues of chronic pain or inflammation. I think fish oil is best for those without fish allergies since the body does not have to "convert" it for use like it must do with plant based oils. Additionally, many of the plant-based sources of essential fatty acids have a lot of omega 6 and 9. Most Americans already consume too much of these, and in excess these can cause inflammation. If you opt to use fish oil, make sure it is heavy metal free (mercury, lead, cadmium, etc.).

        - • Add flaxseed (ground), pumpkin seeds and walnuts. These can help reduce arachidonic acid, and therefore inflammation.

        - • Eat foods and spices that can block enzymes known to increase pain and inflammation. These are known as anti-inflammatory foods. They include ginger, cayenne pepper, turmeric, green tea, red wine, pineapples, avocados, garlic, onions and fish oil.

♣ **Nightshades and Arthritis:** If there is an underlying arthritic condition there are several additional foods that are thought to be detrimental. They are generally known as nightshades. The most commonly consumed nightshades include white potatoes, tomatoes, eggplant, peppers (any kind) and paprika. I have seen miraculous results when people afflicted with arthritis completely eliminate these foods from their diet.

In contrast, Oriental medicine considers cherries (especially black cherries) to be the best food therapy for arthritis. Turmeric and prickly pear is also extremely beneficial. These interventions can be helpful to someone who is experiencing arthritis, while at the same time trying to prevent or manage overuse symptoms.

♣ **pH Balance:** Your body should be slightly more alkaline than acidic. Ideally, it should remain within a range of 6.8 and 7.5. However many, if not most, Americans fall well below that level. The ramifications of being in a chronic acidic state are significant. It impacts every system in the body. If the pH levels are too low, a condition called acidosis results. Your body's pH affects your electrolyte levels, which in turn affect the assimilation of needed nutrients. Eventually this can cause weakening of the body, provide a medium in which unhealthy cells proliferate, and make it difficult for the body to heal.

o The chief reason your body becomes acidic is the intake of acid-forming foods and drinks. Some common culprits include coffee, tea, milk, soda, meat, refined sugar and fruit juices. Some common foods that help alkalinize the body include celery, raw spinach, broccoli, lemons (although they are acidic, they leave an alkaline "residue"), maple syrup, green vegetables and apples.

You can easily test your urinary pH balance using test strips purchased in your local health food store, pharmacy or off the internet.

Food and Emotions: How you eat can also impact your stress levels and emotions, thus dramatically affecting your experience of pain.

There are several things I advise my patients to eat, or avoid if they are dealing with high levels of stress in their lives. What you eat affects your brain chemistry, which of course directly affects how you feel. Some considerations follow:

- **Dark Chocolate:** My patients are sometimes surprised when I tell them that a *little* dark chocolate might be good for them to add to their diet, especially if they are dealing with depression. It stimulates a variety of "feel good" chemicals and hormones that help elevate mood. It actually helps to change brain chemistry. Benefits can be seen within a few minutes to a few days, depending on the severity of the depression.

  Most people think of chocolate as the epitome of junk food. Actually, *dark* chocolate can provide some significant, proven health benefits. Dark chocolate (I usually recommend at least 65% organic dark chocolate) is chock full of flavonoids, which are natural antioxidants. Antioxidants help slow down the aging process, as well as reduce damaging free radicals that can lead to various diseases, including heart disease, and slow down the body's ability to heal itself. Additionally, flavonoids help lower "bad" cholesterol, and along with cocoa phenols, can assist in reducing blood pressure.

  So how much is beneficial to eat? And is milk chocolate just as good? Studies indicate only need a small amount of dark chocolate a day can help elevate mood. My experience with patients is that a little dark chocolate can work remarkably fast. It is important to eat only a little. More is not better. Even dark chocolate is high in calories, fat and sugar. Too much can lead to weight gain and other complications. Chocolate also has some mild stimulants that are not helpful in large amounts. Milk chocolate does not have the same health benefits as dark chocolate and is often higher in fat and sugar content.

- **Complex Carbohydrates:** Along with protein, complex carbs serve an important function in the production of serotonin in the brain. Serotonin is pivotal to help elevate mood. Complex carbs include *whole* grains, beans, lentils, and starchy vegetables (although white potatoes are not the best source). I have seen people start to feel significantly better within a week of drastically increasing their intake of complex carbs. As a side note, complex carbohydrates are *not* bad for you, nor do they cause weight gain. Most weight gain from carbs is due to the consumption of refined, processed carbohydrates rather than the whole, unprocessed food.

o **Protein:** Protein is essential for the production of serotonin and other chemicals in the body that are necessary for healthy emotions. A good rule of thumb for calculating serving size is that your protein serving should be about the size of your open palm.

It is important to be especially mindful of how much protein you ingest if you suffer from depression accompanied by anger and irritation. This may indicate that you are ingesting too much protein without enough complex carbohydrates, leading to an over abundance of dopamine and norepinephrine which can lead to these types of emotions. In this situation it can be helpful to increase the consumption of complex carbohydrates and reduce the amount of protein ingested.

o **Eliminate excitotoxins:** As mentioned above, excitotoxins hyper-stimulate and excite neurons. As well as impacting your experience of pain, they are thought by many to affect the emotions as well. I have seen tremendous improvements in the emotional health of patients who stopped or significantly reduced their intake of excitotoxins. The most common ones that I see people using are artificial sweeteners and Monosodium Glutamate (MSG).

o **Avoid smoking:** Though it is not a food, smoking is something that you take into your body which can impact your risk of overuse injury. When you smoke, you absorb carbon monoxide and nicotine into your body. These substances reduce the supply of oxygen to your body and brain. Although smoking can negatively impact your body in a variety of ways, it can also affect your risk of overuse injury for three reasons:

▪ First, brain function is diminished when there is insufficient oxygen. This affects concentration and processing abilities. This can add tremendous stress to someone engaged in activities that require these abilities.

- Second, because muscle tissue needs oxygen in order to function in a healthy manner, smoking will increase the risk of injury, along with compromising the body's ability to heal.

- Third, smoking is a vaso-constrictor and so reduces the circulation and availability of oxygen to your cells.

o **Caffeine:** Caffeine can potentially increase pain levels in the body. Because it is a nervous system stimulant it tends to cause increased tension in the muscles. Increased muscle tension equals increased pain.

o **Supplements:** In general, I believe supplements are a good idea if used properly. I have also seen much misuse of supplements. While, I think your body was intended to garner the nutrients it needs from the foods you eat, I also acknowledge that the world is not as it once was. Soil is depleted. The world is contaminated with pollutants that permeate the air, water, food and environment. Stress levels, for many, run chronically high. Since all of these things increase your need for vitamins and minerals, I think a daily supplement is helpful.
I will not describe specific amounts here, since individual needs vary, however what I typically recommend for most adults is:

- A *very good* daily whole food vitamin and mineral supplement. I prefer a supplement made from whole, concentrated food.

- Fish oil (heavy metal free) *unless allergic, sensitive or on blood thinners (usually 1000-3000 grams)

- Alpha-lipoic acid and acetyl-L-carnitine. This combination is wonderful because it assists the mitochondria (the energy making cells) in creating energy for the body's use.

- Tart cherry juice extract for people with arthritis or other inflammatory disorders (caution for diabetics).

- Turmeric as an anti-inflammatory. Incidentally, there is research to indicate that turmeric may play a significant role in prevention of Alzheimer's. (Caution for those with ulcers or acid reflex)

- Chlorophyll water to help keep the PH balance of the body slightly on the alkaline side. Just a few drops will suffice. Chlorophyll can be purchased at your local health food store. One caution with using chlorophyll drops is that it can cause loose stools if you use too much. Just drop the amount back until your stools are formed and easily passed.

Nutrition and Oriental Medicine: Nutritional intervention to assist in healing is an important aspect of Oriental medicine.[11] Some foods are believed to cause Qi, or energy, to become stuck or blocked in the body. This becomes significant when it is understood that where Qi does not flow, there is pain, and where there is pain, Qi is not flowing.

Foods that can cause a stagnation of Qi are:

- Greasy foods

- Excessive dairy, especially cheese

- Cold food and drinks

- Refined foods and sugar

So next time you sit down to a meal, consider making it a pain-free one... and bon appetite!

Chapter 10

Self Care Using Acupressure and Self-Massage

Oriental medicine can be a powerful modality for self care. Learning these techniques is an empowering way to take control of your own health. However, **self-treatment is *not* intended to replace appropriate and necessary medical treatment**. It can, however, effectively supplement any medical intervention. Acupressure and self-massage is a powerful preventive strategy, as well as helping you manage symptoms resulting from overuse.

The effectiveness of the treatments and the number of sessions that may be required depends on how long you have had the injury, how severe it is, your current health status and your lifestyle. If you have a longstanding, chronic condition, repeated treatments over a long period of time may be required. If your symptoms are mild and recent, results may be fast and more dramatic. If your condition is permanent, acupressure and self-massage may be helpful to mediate pain and stress.

Acupressure and self-massage have many significant functions including:

- ♣ **Reduces stress**

- ♣ **Releases physical muscle tension**

- ♣ **Increases blood and Qi circulation**

- ♣ **Dissipates energy blocks**

- ♣ **Stimulates production of white blood cells, thus enhancing immune function**

- ♣ **Releases natural painkillers**

- ♣ **Improves mental function**

- ♣ **Stabilizes and relaxes joints**

- ♣ **Strengthens tendons**

- ♣ **Helps the body heal faster**

♣ **Enhances performance**

♣ **Minimizes future injuries**

General acupressure and self-massage strategies: Following are some helpful suggestions on how to use acupressure and self-massage:

♣ Massage only to the intensity of 3 out of 10. Many people think "more is better." In reality massage or acupressure that is too aggressive can exacerbate things at worst, and be ineffective at best. It is possible that the muscle tissue may rebound and spasm, or cut off the flow of Qi with an overly aggressive approach. Massaging at an intensity level of 3 out of 10 is strong enough to be effective and yet not too forceful to be harmful.

♣ Massage each point for approximately 30 seconds on each side two to three times a day. Too much massage can lead to local bruising and excessive tenderness.

♣ Continue to breathe normally. Breathing allows and encourages the free flow of Qi. Ceasing to breathe normally can result in an increase in physical tension and stagnant Qi.

Tui Na Self Massage: Tui Na is a system of body work that has been performed as an integral part of Oriental medicine for thousands of years. Tui means to "push" and Na means "lift and squeeze." Learning the basics of this time honored system can be helpful because it empowers you with a wonderful tool for self-care.[12] Tui Na bodywork promotes muscle and joint health and mobility.

♣ **Tui Na includes eight primary massage techniques:**

  o **Tui:** Pushing

  o **Na:** Pulling or dragging

  o **An:** Pressing

  o **Tao:** Pinching

- o **Nie:** Kneading

- o **Nipping:** Pressing with nail

- o **Moa:** Rubbing

- o **Pai:** Tapping

There are myriad ways in which Tui Na can be used to help in the prevention and management of overuse injury. Some I have found particularly helpful include:

- ♣ **Every morning:**

    - o **Pai** (tap) the thymus. The thymus is located just behind your breast bone, just above your chest. If you tap firmly about 20 times on the breastbone it can help to stimulate the thymus gland. The intensity should be firm, but not painful.

        The thymus gland is integral to the functioning of other hormonal glands in the endocrine system. I have found that thumping the thymus each morning helps to "wake up" the thymus gland, increases energy and helps to support the endocrine system.

        This technique would be contra-indicated for anyone with heart problems.

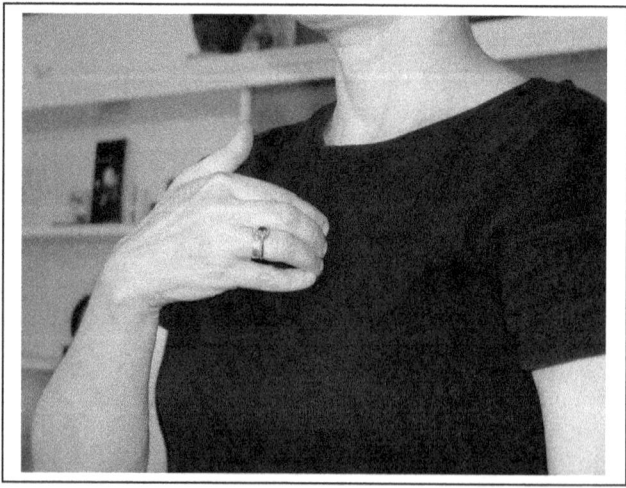

o **Pai** (tap) very gently with fists or cupped hands the outside of your body, from top to bottom, then the inside of your arms and legs from bottom to top.

The abdomen and head should be excluded in this technique and is contra-indicated if on blood thinners or if you bruise easily, and should be avoided on any region of the body that is injured.

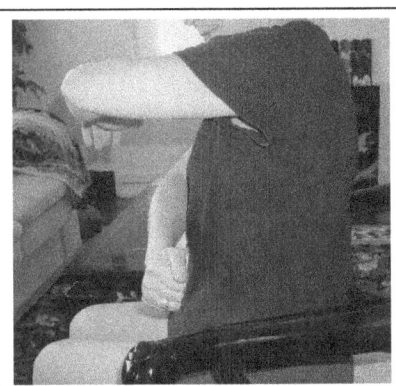 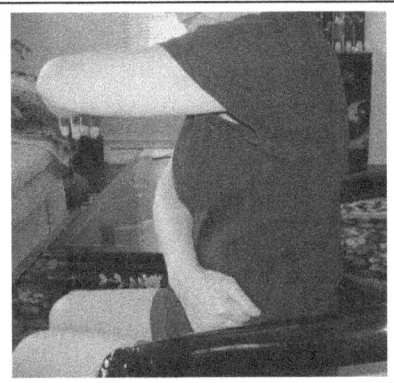

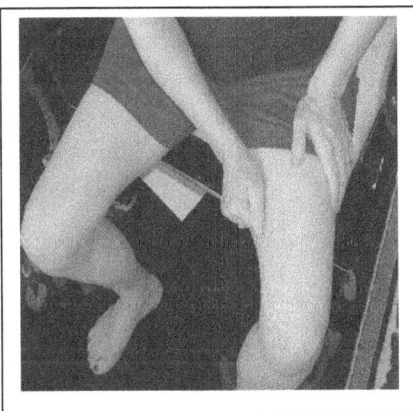 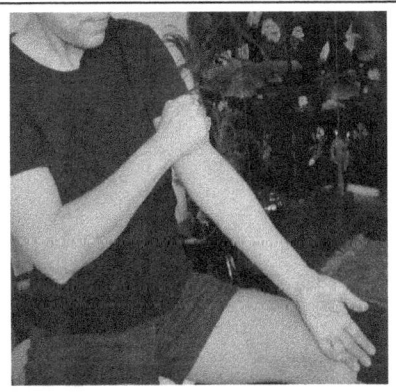

♣ **After meals:**

o **Moa** (rub) your stomach in clockwise circles to stimulate digestion. This is important since the muscles and sinews need nutritional support for the demands repetitive motions place on the body.

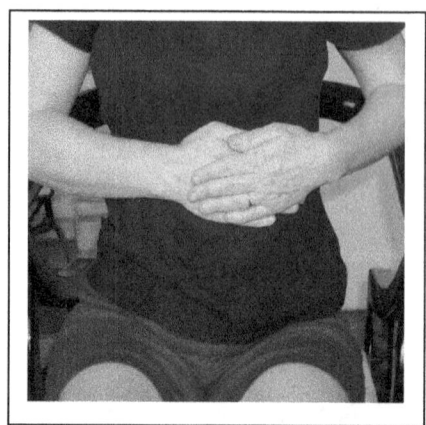

♣ **At night:**

○ **Hold forehead with one palm and base of skull with the other while lying down.** While this is not really a Tui Na technique, I have found it very helpful in reducing stress. When you experience stress a significant amount of blood floods to the back of your head where the limbic system, or the "emotional" brain is located. Placing your hands on the back of your head and on your forehead at the same time keeps some of the blood in the fore-brain, the part that is more focused on logic and reasoning. Basically it helps to balance the reasoning center and the emotional centers of the brain.

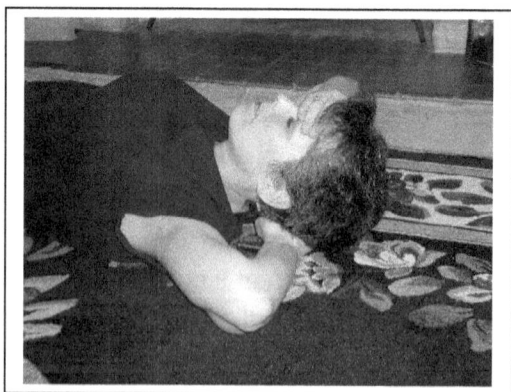

- **Soak feet in hot water for 15 minutes prior to bed.** The temperature should be comfortably warm but not scalding. This helps to bring the energy down and out of the head. It is extremely helpful for insomnia, especially if you have trouble sleeping because you can't "turn your brain off."

♣ **General Daily Regimen:**

- **Na** (pull/drag) fingers from crown, down the side of your head to the neck.

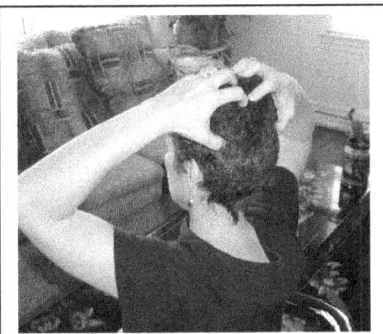 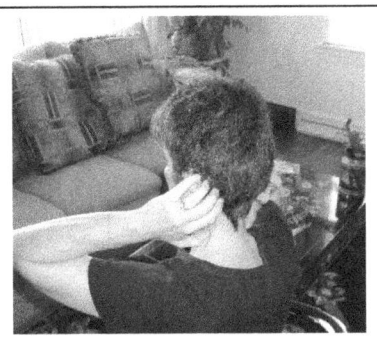

- **Na** (pull/drag) fingers, starting on the forehead between the eyes, moving outward to the temples.

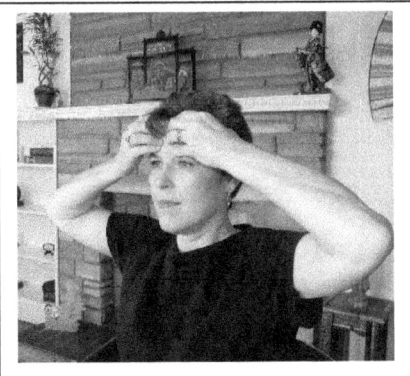 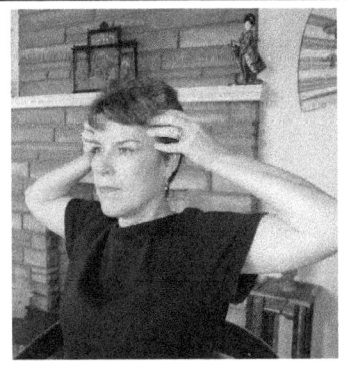

- **Na** (pull/drag) facial muscles and sinuses in a downward movement with fingers.

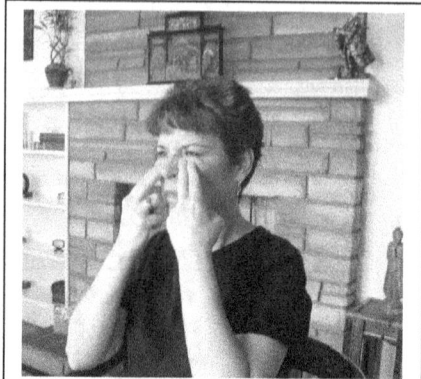
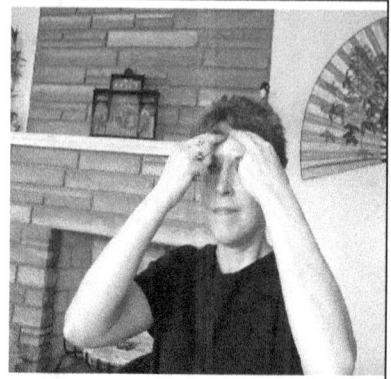

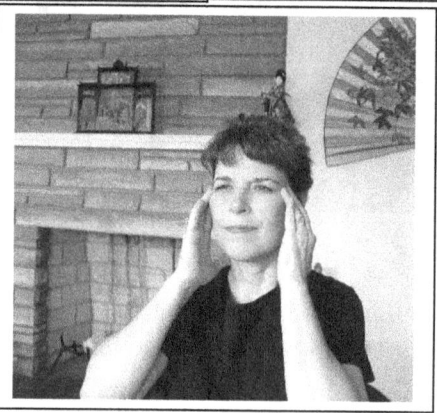

- **Cup closed hands over eyes.** Do not apply any pressure to the eyes with the hands.

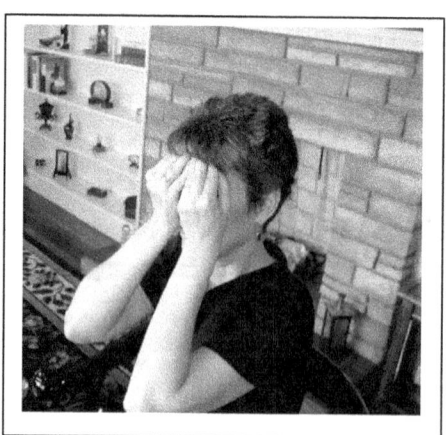

- **Nie** (knead) your ears.

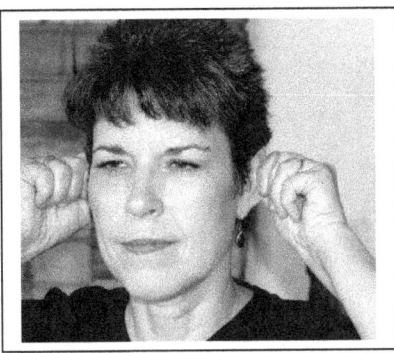

- **Nie** (knead) the nape of the neck using heel of hand. This is done by cupping the entire back of the neck with your palm, then using the heel of the hand to massage. To do both sides, you will need to change hands.

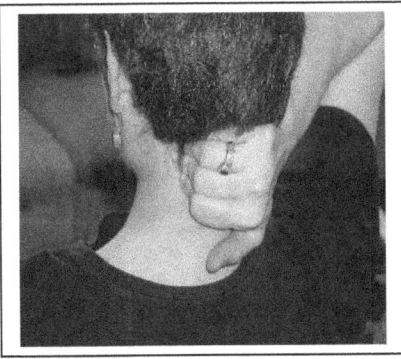

- **Na** (pull/drag) fingers from back of shoulders to front.

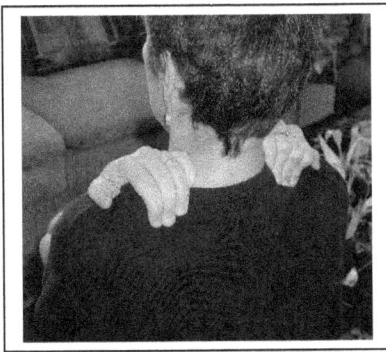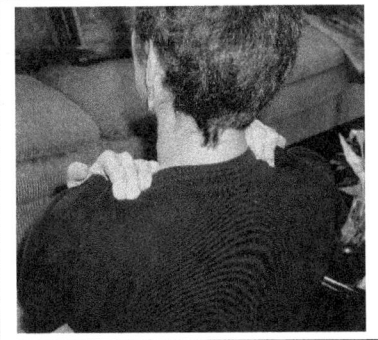

- **Pai** (tapping) shoulders lightly using tips of fingers or brush bristles. This helps to break up stuck Qi and allow for its free flow. Often people experience significant relief from tight shoulders using this technique.

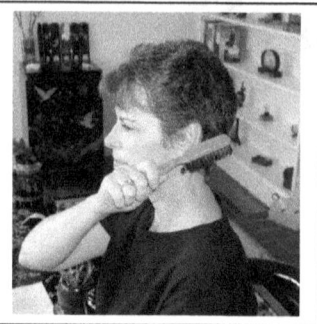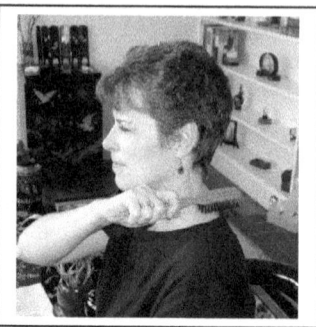

- o **Tui** (push) and **Nie** (knead) arms working from shoulder to hands.

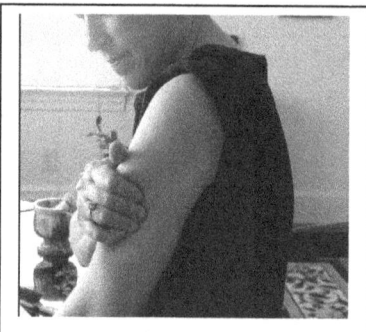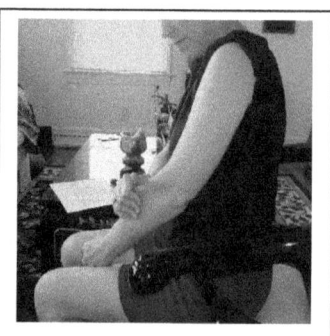

- o **Tao** (pinch) and **Nie** (knead) hands. Sometimes this can be done with oil or lotion.

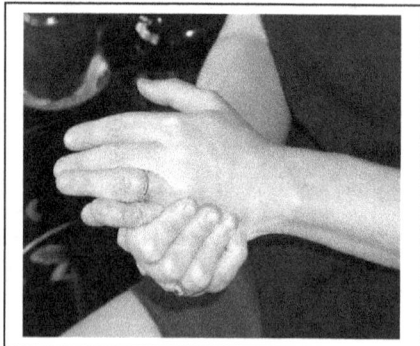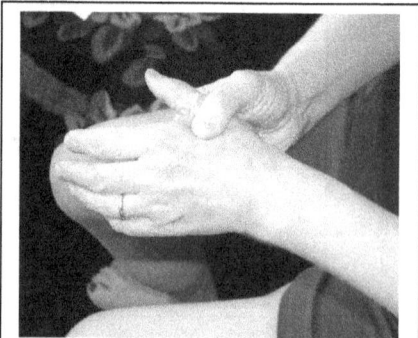

- **Gently grasp shoulder and arm muscles and gently shake.** I have found that gently holding and shaking a muscle is the fastest way to get it to relax. Within just a few seconds there is often a significant release.

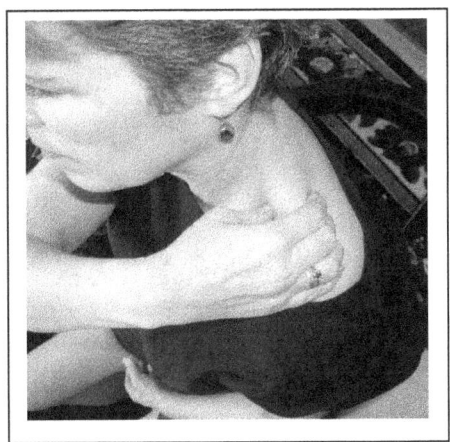

- **Nie** (knead) back muscles and buttocks. Sometimes I recommend people use tennis balls for this. Unless it is painful you may be able to lie down on the balls. Sometimes you can tie two tennis balls in a pair of knee highs with a knot between the balls, place them on a wall and lean into them with your back, while moving your body up and down.

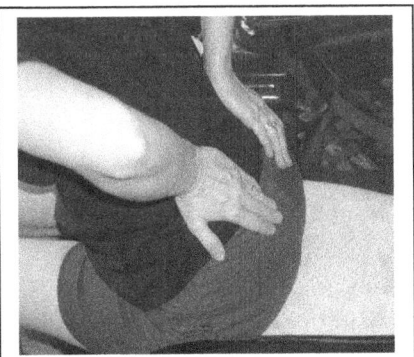 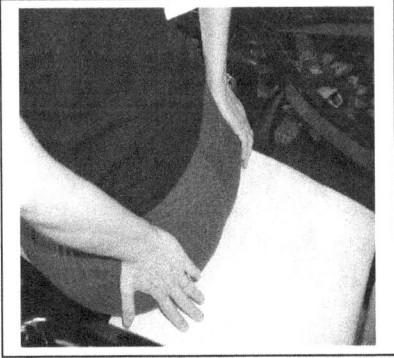

- **An** (press) and **Nie** (knead) legs working from your hips to your feet.

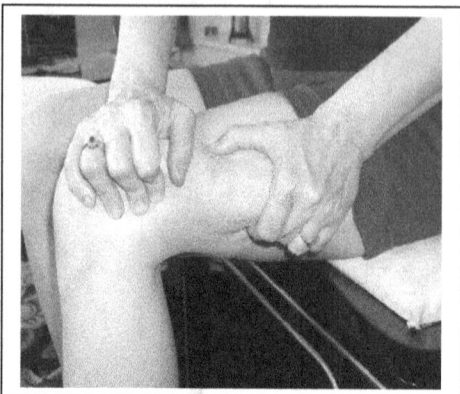 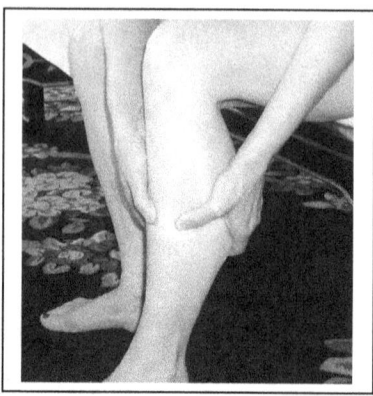

- **Nie** (knead) foot. Some parts of the foot are easier to massage if you link your fingers between your toes and use the palm of your hand.

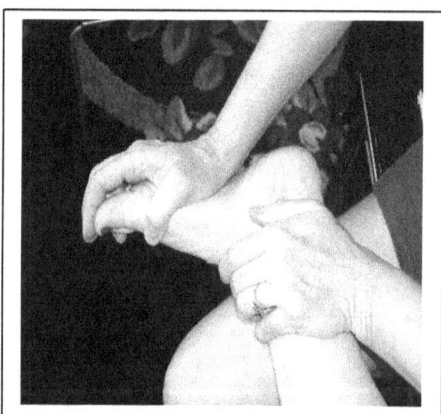 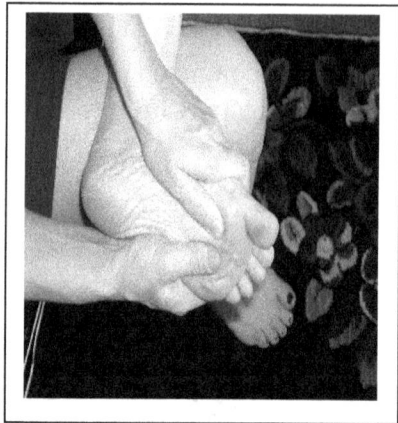

Mirror points: Mirror points are points on the *opposite* extremities from the side of the body experiencing symptoms. For example, if someone comes to me with wrist pain, I may treat their wrist by inserting an acupuncture needle in the ankle on the opposite side. This type of treatment is extremely effective and can be done with massage as well. In order to treat mirror points:

♣ **Determine area of pain**

- ♣ **Identify which extremity should be massaged in order to treat the area of pain.** The corresponding areas are (See Figure 3):
  - o Hip/ankle
  - o Shoulder/ankle
  - o Shoulder/hip
  - o Knee/elbow
  - o Knee/knee
  - o Wrist/ankle

Figure 3

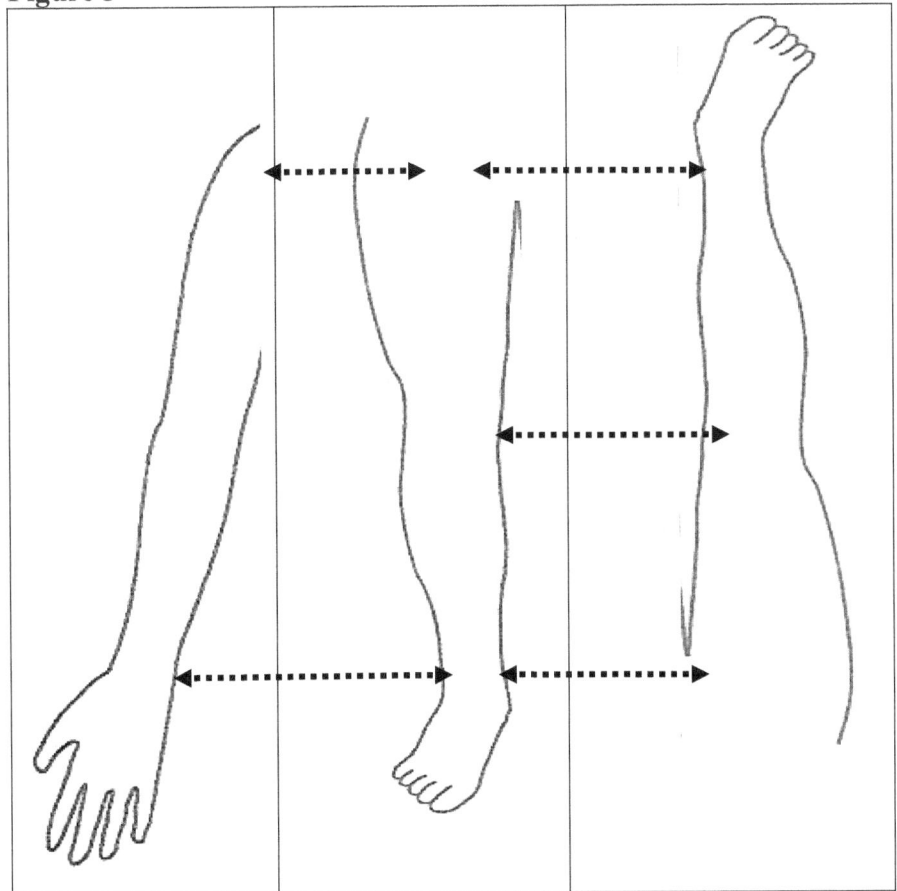

- ♣ **Always treat the opposite side of the body**

♣ **The extremity you will be massaging represents the one being treated.** For example, if the pain is on the thumb side of the right wrist, then massage the big toe side of the left ankle. In other words imagine where the point to treat your wrist would be on your ankle if you ankle were actually your wrist. Basically you "overlay" a template of the extremity that is in pain onto the extremity you are massaging.

♣ **Search for sore areas on the extremity you are massaging.** While you will be able to identify the general area to target for massage by eyeballing it, the tender points are the specific areas to be massaged.

♣ **Move the extremity around that is experiencing the symptoms while simultaneously massaging the limb on the opposite side to get the desired effect.**

♣ **Continue stimulating the point and moving the limb for one-two minutes and then move to another point.**

Hand Micro System: There are a variety of micro systems in acupuncture; however, I want to focus on the micro system of the hand. It can be a wonderful tool for self care. The areas of the hand that are germane for upper extremity overuse are the middle fingers and ring fingers. The middle finger represents the head, neck, shoulders and scapular regions. The ring finger represents the hand, wrist, elbow and shoulder areas. The palm aspect is the front of the body and the back of the hand is the back of the body. It is very important to note that, unlike mirror points, hand micro system points always treat the same side. This means that if the right wrist is hurting, you treat points on the right ring finger. The same principles on how to find the specific sore points with mirror points should be followed here. The only difference is that the same side is treated. Some helpful hints are:

♣ The first joint (closest to the tip of the finger) on the middle finger represents the junction between the head and neck. Often this is a great place to treat when there is neck pain.

♣ The area between the first and second joint of the middle finger is the neck.

- The scapular region is represented by the area between the second and last joint of the middle finger.

- The first joint (closest to the tip) of the ring finger represents the wrist.

  o The second joint of the ring finger corresponds to the elbow.

  o The last joint of the ring finger is the shoulder joint, so the webbing between the last joint of the ring and middle fingers is the area of the trapezius, or shoulder muscles.

Helpful Massage Points: (Note: the abbreviations assigned to the points on figure 4 (e.g. GB20, SJ3, etc.) refer to the identity of the energy channel and the specific point on that channel. So GB20 would refer to the twentieth point along the Gall Bladder energy channel. (For the purposes of this book that level of depth will not be explored and is not necessary to locating and utilizing the points for the purpose of self care.)

See Figure 4 on page 77 for graphic depiction of point location. Point descriptions and explanations are also listed below. Generally you will find the points will be slightly tender. There may even be a small depression where the point is found.

Measurements are designated by Cun (an ancient measurement). One Cun is equivalent to the measurement from the tip of your thumb to the first knuckle. Cun are used because one person's body proportions will be different from another person's.

Self treatment using acupressure points:

NECK:

- **GB20:** On the nape, in the two depressions at the base of the skull below the occipital area.

- **GB39:** On the lateral (outside) aspect of the calf, 3 cun above the tip of the outside ankle bone, in front of the border of the fibula bone.

* **SI3:** When making a loose fist the point is found at the end of the crease on the side of your hand near the little finger.

* **UB60:** On the foot, directly behind the outside ankle bone, in the depression between the ankle bone and the Achilles tendon. (note: This point is contra-indicated for pregnant women.)

* **SJ5:** On the back of the forearm (not palm side), two cun above the wrist between the bones on the arm.

SHOULDER:

* **SJ5:** On the back of the forearm (not palm side), two cun above the wrist between the bones on the arm.

* **LI4:** On the back of the hand, on a sore spot in the webbing between the 1st (index) finger and the thumb. (note: This point is contra-indicated for pregnant women.)

* **ST12:** In the midpoint of the hollow above the clavicle, 4 cun from the midline of the body. (note: This point is contra-indicated for pregnant women.)

* **ST38:** On the front aspect of the lower leg, 8 cun below the knee, one finger-breadth (middle finger) to the outside of the shinbone.

* **GB21:** On the trapezius part of the shoulder, directly above the nipple. This is usually the highest point of the trapezius muscle. (note: This point is contra-indicated for pregnant women)

* **LI15 and SJ14:** These points are found on the shoulder joint. They are two depressions right on the shoulder joint.

ELBOW:

* **SJ5:** On the back of the forearm (not palm side), two cun above the wrist between the bones on the arm.

* **LI4:** On the back of the hand, on a sore spot in the webbing between the 1st (index) finger and the thumb. (note: This point is contra-indicated for pregnant women.)

* **SI8:** This point is found in the depression on the "funny bone" of the elbow.

* **LI11:** With the elbow bent, the point is at the end of the crease on the outside aspect of the arm at the elbow.

* **LI12:** With the elbow bent the point is on the outside aspect of the arm, 1 cun above LI11, on the border of the arm bone.

* **LU5:** On the crease of the elbow, in the depression just on the outside aspect of the large tendon.

WRIST:

* **ST36:** On the front aspect of the lower leg, 3 cun below the bottom of the knee, one fingerbreadth to the outside of the shinbone.

* **SP5:** In the depression below and just to the front of the inside ankle bone.

* **GB40:** In the depression below and just to the front of the outside ankle bone.

* **PC7:** Directly in the middle of the wrist crease, on the palm side of the wrist.

* **LI5:** On the thumb side of the wrist in the large depression at the base of the thumb on the side of the wrist.

* **SJ4:** On the crease on the back aspect of the wrist, in the depression on the little finger side of the tendon. This point is just off center from the midpoint of the back of the wrist.

* **SI4 and SI5:** These two points can be found on the little finger side of the wrist. The points are in depressions just below and just above the wrist crease on the side of the wrist.

FINGERS:

♣ **SJ3:** On the back of the hand, in the depression between the ring finger and little finger and just above the knuckles.

♣ **LI3:** When a loose fist is made, this point is in the fleshy depression on the thumb side of the pointer finger.

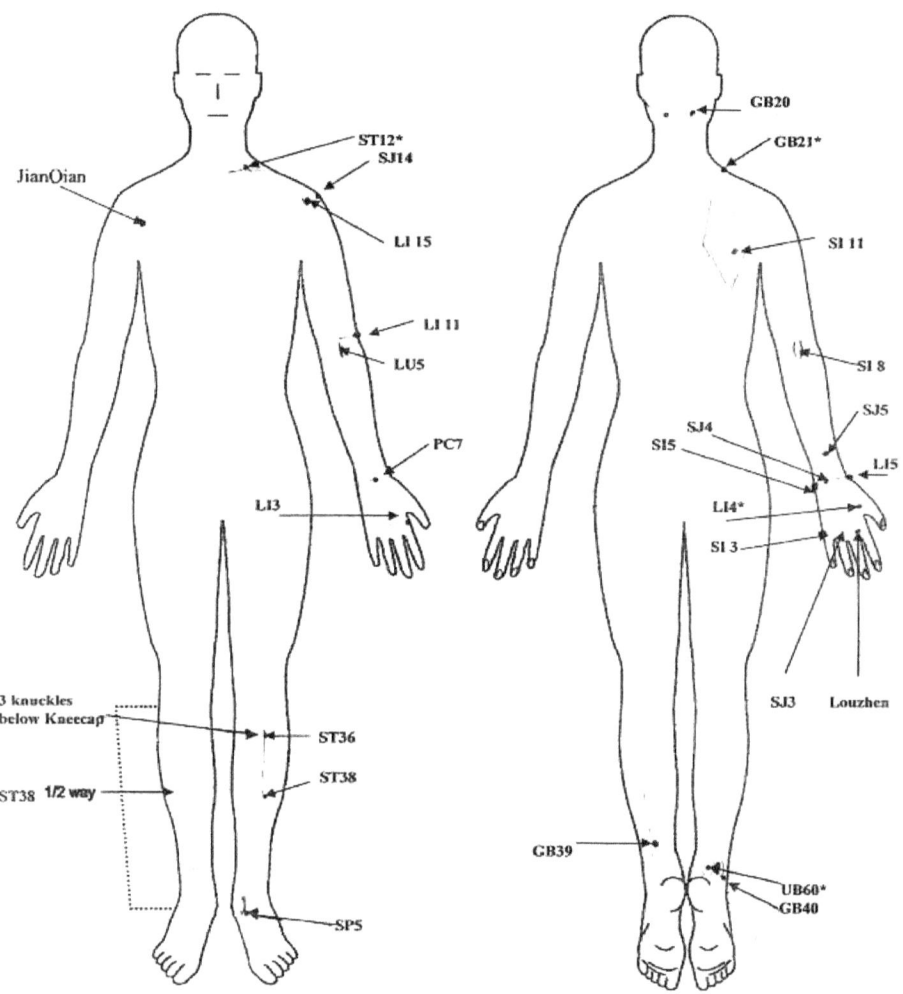

Figure 4 * = **Contraindicated for pregnant women**

Chapter 11

The Yin and Yang of Time

Imagine cruising down the highway on a beautiful spring day in your best friend's fancy new sports car. You converse amiably as he or she skillfully navigates the twists and curves of the road. The scenery is lovely and you are enjoying the company. However, there is a sense of urgency in the air since you are both quite late. As you chat your eyes move past - and then back to - the gas gauge. It's on empty. "Uh, I think you need some gas," you say. To your great surprise your friend responds with, "Well, I don't have time to stop for gas. I'm too busy driving and besides, we're running late!" You are not sure you heard right, so you try again. "Yeah, but we don't have enough gas to get there", you offer. "It's on empty!" Again, the response; "No way I'm stopping! We're already running late, and I am too busy driving to take time to stop for gas."

Most of us would agree that the above scenario doesn't make a lot of sense. Refusing to stop for gas all but guarantees that not only will they not arrive to their destination on time, but that they may not arrive at all. Yet this is the way many people live their lives. I often hear people say they are too busy to take time out of their lives to rest or meditate, or just to sit for a short time in stillness. Great value is placed on doing, achieving and activity, while ceasing the *doing* and simply *being* is given little credence. Sometimes people even feel guilty if they do stop all their activity and just do nothing for a while.

In Oriental medicine everything has a Yin and a Yang aspect. A balance of each is necessary in order for there to be harmony and balance. Yin is a more restful, quiet, yielding type of energy, while Yang energy is more active, dynamic, and forceful. Each must be balanced by the other. Too much rest and quiet time (Yin energy) can lead to lethargy, boredom and stagnation of creative energy. It may also 'snuff out' some of the fire of the Yang energy. Too much activity and *doing* (Yang energy) can lead to burnout, fatigue and overall stressful feelings. It may also 'burn up' some of the Yin energy, leading to illness.

Many people live lives that are not in balance, and yet are surprised when things stop working, or when they "run out of gas'. But systems, including the human body, need balance in order to function optimally. This includes the need for balance between rest and activity, stillness and motion, and meditation and doing.

The benefits of meditation and sitting in stillness are well known. Many research studies over the years have demonstrated this. Some of the benefits of meditation include:

- Improved concentration
- A reduction in feelings of stress
- Improved sleep
- Lower blood pressure
- Better personal relationships
- Overall improved health

It is important to *make* the time for meditation and quietness everyday. Doing so affords the opportunity to get centered and recoup energy. It prevents you from "running out of gas" and allows you to approach all your activities from a more balanced perspective. Just imagine what a day would be like if you felt completely rested, with plenty of energy reserves with which to approach your activities! Or what a day would feel like if you were engaged and active in a balanced way.

It can be helpful to assess whether you need more Yang or more Yin activity in your daily schedule. If you feel you have little or no time to relax, then you probably need to add some Yin activities to your life. If you are a couch potato, then some Yang activities might serve you. And paradoxically, sometimes one is needed in order to support the other. For example, you may need more Yang activity (exercise) in order to sleep better (Yin activity). Or you may need more Yin activity (sleep and meditation time) in order to have the resources to support the Yang activities in your daily life.

It can also be instructive to consider the balance within the Yin and Yang aspects, respectively. For example, if someone meditates 2 hours everyday, but also only *sleeps* two hours every day, then there may not be a balance *within* the Yin aspect of life's activities. If someone works 16 hour days doing computer programming, but gets no physical exercise, then there may be no balance within the Yang aspect. So there must be balance *within* each aspect as well as *between* the two aspects.

Stopping for gas actually facilitates your ability to get where you're going. So too, slowing down, meditating or being contemplative, actually increases your effectiveness in what you want to accomplish.

Making time to "fill up" and restore your energy, and balancing Yin and Yang activities is essential for a balanced and happy life. You actually waste time and compromise productivity when you don't do it.

Chapter 12
Work Stations

Footrests:

When you have to sit at a station for a long period of time, such as in a call center or office, there should be a footstool at your workstation. The footrest should allow for independent height and angle adjustments. This will allow each person to find the position of the legs and feet best for them. Thighs should ideally be parallel to the floor or only slightly angled down when seated properly.

It is important to take care not to use the footrest to compensate for a chair that is too high. Sometimes people try to use footrests to substitute for a lower chair and/or workstation. When a person inappropriately uses a footrest to compensate for inappropriate chair or workstation heights, awkward leg postures may result. Make sure the foot doesn't rest on sharp or hard edges. Big footrests give more choice of leg posture. Footrests should be stable enough to stay in place but easy to move with the feet and legs to reposition if needed.

Chairs:

There are several features that are important to consider with chairs. Generally, if a chair is intended to meet the needs of a number of different body sizes and shapes it is helpful to have a wide variety of options and features. Some helpful features include:

- **Seat height adjustability-** Pneumatic adjustability is easier to use than mechanical. This is important in order to compensate for people of different heights and for easy and fast adjustments.

- **Seat depth adjustability -** This changes the front-to-back depth of the seat either by backrest in-out adjustability or a sliding seat pan. A shorter seat pan allows smaller people to use the chair's backrest, while a deeper one feels more stable to taller individuals.

- **Backrest angle adjustability-**The ability to change the angle of the backrest.

- ♣ **Chair tilt:** The angle of the entire seat relative to the floor. A reclined chair transfers some upper-body weight to the backrest of the chair.

- ♣ **Seat pan angle adjustability:** Changing the forward-back angle of the seat. This feature provides forward tilt, in which the thighs slope downward.

- ♣ **Armrests:** I would not recommend armrests at all. People often use the arms to rest the elbow which can instigate elbow pain. Additionally, chairs with arms seem to contribute to higher risk ergonomics. I have also found that when people rest their arms on the chair arm it pushes their entire upper arm and shoulder upward, increasing tension and static loading in the shoulder region.

- ♣ **Lumbar support:** Helps to minimize the flattening of the lumbar spine when seated. If the lumbar support is not adjustable though, different sized people will have the "bump" hit them at different places in the back and may cause discomfort.

- ♣ **Backrest height adjustability:** This refers to a change in height of the lumbar support area of the chair backrest. This feature accommodates preferences of different people regarding where and how the lumbar support curve contacts the back.

- ♣ **Lumbar depth adjustability:** This allows for adjustment of the size and sometimes the firmness of the lumbar support curve. Like backrest height adjustability, it accommodates different preferences and body shapes.

Desks:

- ♣ If desks are used they should be height adjustable using an automatic rather than manual mechanism.

Monitors:

- ♣ Optimal distance is 20-30 inches.

♣ Monitor should be directly in front of you (height) and aligned so that the top row of characters on the screen is at or slightly below eye level.

Keyboards:

♣ Keyboards should be positioned such that the elbows are able to remain comfortably positioned near the side of the body. The wrist and hand should maintain a neutral position instead of the wrist bending due to the awkward position of the keyboard. In my opinion it is optimal for the forearms to remain as perpendicular to the ground as possible. This avoids static loading from holding the arms up for extended periods of time for keyboarding. A common error is placing the keyboard too high.

Chapter 13

Making Your Body Your Ally

If you are a person experiencing symptoms of overuse, you may find yourself at times feeling as though you are in an adversarial relationship with your own body. You may even find yourself using language such as "my bad arm" or "my no-good hand." While it can be frustrating when life is so profoundly affected by pain from overuse, it is important to remember that your body is not your enemy. In truth, your body constantly works very hard on your behalf. You are actually "hard-wired" to heal; it is your default programming.

You can, however, significantly impact your ability to heal by how you view and treat your body. If you see your body as an enemy, treat it with neglect, deny it adequate amounts of sleep and rest, feed it food filled with toxins rather than needed nutrients, and get little to no exercise, then you burden your body and healing is compromised. If you view your body as your ally, treat it with compassionate regard, balance your sleep and rest with appropriate levels of activity, and consume nutritious foods and sufficient water, then you support your body's natural propensity to heal.

In my practice of Oriental medicine, I treat many people for overuse injuries. While acupuncture and oriental medicine are quite helpful for a variety of overuse symptoms, the prognosis for each patient also depends on their willingness to befriend their body and attend to its needs. I call this making your body your ally. I have found that there are some crucial factors that are essential in order to make your body your ally. These are:

1. Recognize that your body constantly works on your behalf to heal. It is not against you and it is not your enemy. When you view parts of your body as "bad" or "broken" or "no good," then you automatically create an adversarial relationship with your body. This is not conducive to healing.

    In recent years there has been some ground-breaking research in the area of quantum physics that demonstrates our thoughts impact our capacity to heal.[13] If you send angry, hateful thoughts or sentiments to parts of yourself that are in pain, you only add to that pain. It is not much different than getting angry at a child in pain. Anger will not assuage the child's pain, but most likely will increase his or her anguish. When you experience pain, your body is doing what it is supposed to do; it is letting you know that something is wrong and asking you for help.

2. Take a positive approach with your body and healing. Instead of saying, "my bad arm," try saying "the arm in the process of healing." Ask yourself what you can do to show compassion to the part of your body that is in pain.

3. Honor and support your body by providing it the basic essentials that are required for health. This includes nutritious food, adequate water, moderate exercise and restful sleep.

4. Foster fulfilling and intimate relationships in your life. People who have meaningful relationships live longer, healthier lives.

5. Give your body time to heal if you are experiencing an overuse injury. Making sure you give your body sufficient recovery time to heal from an overuse injury will often prevent long term consequences. It is important to listen and respond to your body's needs. In this way you can become an ally to your body and support it as it heals.

6. Listen to your body as it "talks" to you. If you listen and respond, then you will develop a strong alliance and sense of trust with your body. And your body will trust you because you respond to its needs!

7. **Do not** sacrifice your body on the altar of any job or activity. Build time into your schedule to allow your body time to heal if that is what it needs. Taking care of your body is a primary professional and personal responsibility.

8. Warming up before work or an activity, and cooling down afterward is a gift to your body. It is a gentle and caring way to help your body adjust to the physical demands placed on the body by work and play.

Your body works ceaselessly for your good. Listening to your body and becoming aware of its needs is imperative for good health – however, it is only a first step. Once you have the awareness, then action needs to be taken in order to correct any imbalance. Signals of discomfort communicated by the body are not much different than a good friend and neighbor pounding on your door at 2AM to let you know your house is on fire. If you get mad at the neighbor and turn over and go back to sleep, your house may burn down – with you in it! Your friend is doing you a service by pounding on your door. So too is your body.

Sources:

1. Rochester Institute of Technology (2008, April 19). Sign Language Interpreters at High Ergonomic Risk.

2. Bureau of Labor Statistics, U.S. Department of Labor, Survey of Occupational Injuries and Illnesses (in cooperation with participating State agencies), Reissue date: 2009

3. Stuckless, Avery and T. Alan Hurwitz, eds. 1989. Educational interpreting for deaf students: report of the task force on educational interpreting. New York: National Technical Institute for the Deaf, Rochester Institute of Technology.

4. DeCaro, James J., Michael Feuerstein, and T. Alan Hurwitz. "Cumulative trauma disorders among educational interpreters." American Annals of the Deaf 137 (1992): 288-292

5. Feuerstein, Michael, and Terence E. Fitzgerald. "Bio-mechanical factors affecting upper extremity cumulative trauma disorders in sign language interpreters." Journal of Occupational Medicine 34 (1992): 257-264

6. Lynn S. Bickley. Bates Guide to Physical Examination and History Taking, Eighth Edition, Lippincott Williams and Wilkins, 2002

7. Cumulative Trauma Disorder, Rochester Institute of Technology, 2005

8. Maoshing Ni, The Yellow Emperor's Classic of Medicine: A New Translation of the Neijing Suwen with Commentary, Shambahala Publications, 1995

9. Hyman, Mark M.D. The UltraMind Solution, Scribner Publishing (A division of Simon & Schuster, Inc), 2009

10. L. Zhang, M. Fiala, J. Cashman, et al., Curcuminoids enhance amyloid-ß uptake by macrophages of Alzheimer's disease patients. J Alzheimers Dis, 2006, vol. 10, pp. 1-7

11. Flaws, Bob. The Tao of Healthy Eating, Blue Poppy Press, 7th printing 2005

12. Xu Xiangcau. Chinese Tuina Massage: The Essential Guide to Treating Injuries, Improving Health, and Balancing Qi. YMMA Publication Center, Boston, MA., 2002

Other Resources:

Akabas, S.H., L.B. Gates, and D.E. Galvin. Disability management: A complete guide to reduce costs, increase productivity, meet employee needs, and ensure legal compliance. New York, NY: American Management Association, 1992

Caponigro, Andy. The Miracle of the Breath: Mastering Fear, Healing Illness, and Experiencing the Divine. New World Library, 2005

Cohn, Lester, Rhonda M. Lowry, and Sandra Hart. "Overuse syndromes of the upper extremity in interpreters for the deaf." Orthopedics (1989): 207-209

Crouch, Tammy, and Michael Madden. Carpal Tunnel Syndrome and Overuse Injuries. Berkley: North Atlantic Books, 1992

Cumulative Trauma Disorder – CTD, Published by The Rochester Institute of Technology, 1996

Deadman, Peter, and Baker, Kevin. A Manual of Acupuncture, Journal of Chinese Medicine Publications, 2007

Emmons, Henry and Krantz, Rachel. The Chemistry of Joy, Fireside Publishing, 2006

Feldenkrais, Moshe. Awareness Through Movement: Easy-to-Do Health Exercises to Improve Your Posture Vision Imagination and Personal Awareness, Reprint Edition Paperback (Harper San Francisco; Apr 1 1991

Feuerstein, Michael, and P.F. Hickey. "Ergonomic approaches in the clinical assessment of occupational musculoskeletal disorders." In Handbook of pain assessment, edited by D.C. Turk and R. Melzack, 71-99. New York: Guilford Press, 1992

Feuerstein, Michael. "A multidisciplinary approach to the prevention, evaluation, and management of work disability." Journal of Occupational Rehabilitation 1 (1991): 5-11

Hans-Ulrich Hecker, Angelika Steveling, and Elmar Peuker. Microsystems Acupuncture: The Complete Guide: Ear - Scalp - Mouth - Hand, Thieme International Publishing, 2005

HR World Editors, "The Ultimate Guide to Workstation Ergonomics: 10 Easy Tips," October 1, 2007

Kapchuck, Ted. The Web That Has No Weaver, Contemporary Books, 2000

National Institute of Health. "For Parents: Why Sleep is Important. http://www.nhlbi.nih.gov/health/public/sleep/starslp/parents/whysleep.html

Perricone, Nicholas M.D. The Perricone Promise, Warner Books, 2004

Putz-Anderson, Vern, ed. 1988. Cumulative trauma disorders: a manual for musculoskeletal diseases of the upper limbs. London: Taylor and Francis

Sanderson, Gary. "Repetitive Motion Injury." (videotape). Sign Media, Inc.

Stanford University, http://www.stanford.edu/dept/EHS/prod/general/ergo/

Stone, W.E. "Occupational repetitive strain injuries." Australian Family Physician 13 (1984): 682

University Of Maryland. "Sleep Hygiene: Helpful Hints to Help You Sleep" http://www.umm.edu/sleep/sleep_hyg.html

About The Author:

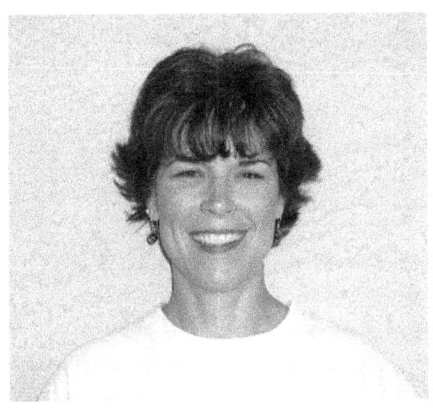

Dr. Diane Gross, DOM (NM), Dipl. OM, L.Ac., HLC, is a Doctor of Oriental medicine (NM), licensed acupuncturist and Holistic Life Coach. Dr. Gross treats many individuals with overuse injury in a highly successful and busy acupuncture clinic in Greensboro, NC. She also serves as a nationally recognized consultant, specializing in providing instruction and diagnostics for people seeking to reduce or manage their risk of interpreting related pain and injury.

Dr. Gross served as Project Coordinator and senior writer in the development of training materials on the prevention and management of interpreting related injury for the National Technical Institute of Technology (NTID) in the early 1990s. Since that time she has continued to provide workshops and assessments for companies across the country. She also brings a unique perspective on self-care using principles based in Oriental medicine, acupressure, self-massage and nutritional interventions.

Dr. Gross is currently the managing practitioner at Stillpoint Acupuncture, located in North Carolina, as well as the owner of TerpHealth_{TM}. She utilizes her extensive knowledge of ergonomics, energy medicine, nutrition and Oriental medicine with her patients and clients with ongoing success.

Dr. Gross can be contacted through her website at **www.TerpHealth.com.** Other books written by Diane include *The Art of Personal Alchemy: Transform Your Emotional Lead into Gold,* and *Sign Safely, Interpret Intelligently: A Guide to the Prevention and Management of Interpreting Related Injury.* She was also senior writer of *Cumulative Trauma Disorder* for the Rochester Institute of Technology.

www.ingramcontent.com/pod-product-compliance
Lightning Source LLC
Chambersburg PA
CBHW072106280526
45788CB00006B/2422